Springer Series on the Teaching of Nursing

Diane O. McGivern, RN, PhD, FAAN, Series Editor
New York University Division of Nursing

Advisory Board: Ellen Baer, PhD, RN, FAAN; Carla Mariano, EdD, RN; Janet A. Rodgers, PhD, RN, FAAN; Alice Adam Young, PhD, RN

Rita Mertig, MS, RNC, CNS, is a professor of nursing at John Tyler Community College in Chester, Virginia. She is coordinator for the third semester which includes maternity nursing, pediatric nursing, and psychiatric/mental health nursing. Mertig teaches maternal-newborn nursing, as well as a health assessment course, test-taking in nursing, and the fluid and electrolyte content in the fundamentals of nursing course. She has taught the diabetes section of the beginning medical-surgical nursing course. She has prior teaching experience in baccalaureate, diploma, and practical nursing settings.

She was graduated from Georgetown University with a bachelor of science in nursing degree and received her master of science degree from the University of California, San Francisco Medical Center, School of Nursing. A clinical specialist, she is certified in maternal-newborn nursing and is also a certified childbirth educator. She contributed chapters to fundamentals of nursing and nursing skills textbooks and wrote the chapter on diabetes in *Nurses Guide to Consumer Health Web Sites*. She has been a reviewer for fundamentals of nursing, nursing skills, and maternity nursing textbooks, as well as for a test bank book.

Shelley F. Conroy, EdD, MS, RN, is currently Dean for Professional and Technical Studies at John Tyler Community College in Chester, Virginia. Until assuming her current position, she served as nursing program coordinator at John Tyler Community College for eight years. She has prior teaching experience in baccalaureate and associate degree settings.

Dr. Conroy received her doctorate in curriculum and instruction from the University of Central Florida, and her master of science and bachelor of science degrees in nursing from Virginia Commonwealth University/Medical College of Virginia.

TEACHING NURSING IN AN ASSOCIATE DEGREE PROGRAM

Rita G. Mertig, MS, RNC, CNS

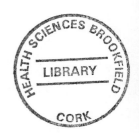

Springer Series on the Teaching of Nursing

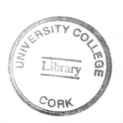

Copyright © 2003 by Springer Publishing Company, Inc.

Springer Publishing Company, Inc.
536 Broadway
New York, NY 10012-3955

Acquisitions Editor: Ruth Chasek
Production Editor: Janice Stangel
Cover design by Joanne E. Honigman

03 04 05 06 07 / 5 4 3 2 1

Library of Congress Cataloging-in-Publication Data

Mertig, Rita G.
    Teaching nursing in an associate degree program / Rita G. Mertig.
       p. ; cm. — (Springer series on the teaching of nursing)
    Includes bibliographical references and index.
    ISBN 0-8261-2004-0
    1. Nursing—Study and teaching (Associate degree) 2. Associate degree nurses. I. Title. II. Springer series on the teaching of nursing (Unnumbered)
    [DNLM: 1. Education, Nursing, Associate. 2. Teaching—methods. WY 18 M575t 2003]
    RT74.5.M47 2003
    610.73'071'1—dc21   2003050614

Printed in the United States of America by Maple-Vail Book Manufacturing Group.

This book is dedicated to my husband, Bob, to my children, Karen and Kelley, and to all the students whom I have had the pleasure of teaching.

R. G. Mertig

Contents

Foreword

*T*eaching Nursing in an Associate Degree Program by Rita Mertig is an important addition to the Springer Series on the Teaching of Nursing. The content is presented in a straightforward manner that will be most useful to those new to AD level education or to new teachers of nursing at any level. It is important to note that while the author draws on her own experience and that of her colleagues who teach in AD programs, many of the principles have applicability across all levels of basic nursing education.

In this book, the author covers the most significant topics central to entry-level nursing education. These include teaching strategies and motivational strategies for all AD nursing students and a chapter devoted to students who fail, with suggestions for helping these students to understand the factors inhibiting their success. Chapter 2, the only contributed chapter in the book, is written by Shelley Conroy, a nurse educator with experience both in nursing education and educational administration at the AD level. As detailed by Conroy, AD prepared nurses now represent the largest percentage of Registered Nurses (RNs) in the United States. In this chapter, Conroy provides basic information about the characteristics of the AD student in nursing. With the increased demand for new nurses, there is the expectation within the nursing education community that AD programs in nursing will expand as more students from diverse backgrounds are recruited into the 2-year programs.

Three chapters included in the book are especially noteworthy. Chapter 4 is focused on socialization of the student into the profession of nursing. Chapter 7 describes the teacher's role as mentor. Chapter 8 serves as an excellent summary chapter, with attention to two key topics: addressing nursing workforce issues through the recruitment of students and their socialization into the nursing role, and the positive influence of teachers in helping to retain nurses within the profession once they have been prepared.

Often individuals recruited to teach in AD programs have excellent clinical skills and a wealth of clinical experiences, but very little teaching experience in either formal classroom or clinical settings. In addition, because of the current shortage of nurse faculty, most often new teachers do not have mentors to guide them through the essentials of the teaching-learning process. They may be left to learn on their own and to engage in "trial and error" approaches. Some rely on the teaching skills that were used by faculty in their own basic nursing program, yet techniques of teaching nursing from five, ten, or 20 years ago may not work with the students of today. Students in AD programs today often have competing life demands. They often are adults with family and job responsibilities. Often, nursing is a second career for the AD student. Thus, the teaching techniques required of the faculty member might be quite different.

Mertig has years of experience as a nursing educator in a wide range of educational programs, from practical nursing programs to baccalaureate nursing programs. All of her teaching experiences have been with students new to the profession of nursing. The practical advice that she offers to other teachers is refreshing; it will be welcomed by new inexperienced nurse educators as well as those who have been teaching for years, but are frustrated by the increasing demands of the educator role. Mertig's advice to nurse educators is basic, but extremely important. She begins by helping educators to understand their own attitudes, motivations, and teaching behaviors. She points out that as teachers of future generations of professional nurses, nurse educators face high expectations. She also reinforces the fact that a commitment to excellence in developing their skills as nurse educators can yield significant rewards. The faculty will see the students' confidence and competence grow, as they learn and hone their professional nursing skills.

One of the best parts of this book is the inclusion of the "how to" tips, many of which are based on Mertig's personal experiences as a nurse educator. In addition to the examples that she includes for motivating and teaching students, Mertig has included assessment instruments and handy summaries of key elements for certain situations (e.g., elements of a course on test taking) that have been advantageous to her in her teaching.

New and experienced nurse educators will find helpful hints, useful motivational techniques, and key strategies for basic nursing education in this handbook. And, importantly, all of the author's advice is presented in the context of meeting the needs of the students, the profession, and the communities served by the AD nursing programs.

Joyce J. Fitzpatrick, PhD, MBA, RN, FAAN
Elizabeth Brooks Ford Professor of Nursing
and former Dean of Nursing
Frances Payne Bolton School of Nursing
Case Western Reserve University, Cleveland, OH

Figures, Tables, and Boxes

Acknowledgments

I would like to thank formally the following people who made it possible to write this book:

Dr. Ursula Springer, who gave me the opportunity to write this book after meeting with me only once and Ruth Chasek, my contact person at Springer Publishing, who was so generous with her time, advice, and encouragement.

My friend and mentor, Dr. Joyce Fitzpatrick, who introduced me to Dr. Springer, encouraged me to write this book, and wrote the foreword. Her faith in me was empowering and kept me going. Her editing and suggestions were invaluable.

My family, who gave of their time generously and were always willing to rearrange planned family events to suit my writing schedule; I owe them my sanity. My adult daughters, Karen and Kelley, generously gave me the benefit of their wisdom in editing several chapters. Kelley typed and retyped tables and boxes and helped with the general organization and consistency of the book. My husband, Bob, took over all the cooking, cleaning, and grocery shopping chores so I could pursue my goal of completing this manuscript.

My boss, Dr. Shelley Conroy, who consented to write the second chapter, despite her recent promotion and added responsibilities; I am very grateful. In addition, I would like to thank Chanda Rainey, our newest faculty member, who agreed to read the first several chapters. Her positive comments about how the manuscript directed her journey toward becoming an effective community college nursing educator invigorated me as I struggled to complete the last chapters.

My friend and typist, Donna Davis, who put up with my handwriting and my many arrows and odd directions; thanks for saving me a lot of time and energy. Lastly, my students, who helped me to learn, over the years, how to help them meet their educational and professional goals. They shared their stories, their hopes, and their difficulties, and allowed me to share my vision for them. To the many who have returned to tell us of their career successes, I am grateful.

Rita G. Mertig

1

Introduction

Some individuals come to their faculty position knowing little if any-thing about the principles of teaching and learning. Many who have been in a faculty role for several years may know only those approaches to teaching or evaluating learning that they experienced themselves as students or to which their senior colleagues introduced them when they first started in the role (NLN Position Statement, September, 2001, paragraph 4).

For most of my professional career, I have been teaching nursing in a variety of educational settings, including a baccalaureate program, a practical nursing program, a diploma school program, and, for the last 17 years, in an associate degree nursing program. During my tenure teaching at various levels of nursing preparation, I have come to realize that there are typical commonalities and distinct differences between the student populations in each program. Over the years, I have also become acutely aware of the changing attributes of the students in the community college in general and the nursing program in particular. This observation is not new to anyone who has worked with this population. However, these students remain dedicated to achieving success in nursing, despite the many educational and logistical problems that they face.

I began thinking about this book many years ago, when I discovered that my master's degree in teaching nursing, my clinical practice, and my prior teaching experience in a baccalaureate nursing program had not prepared me to teach in an associate degree nursing program. These students were not 18 to 22 years of age. Most did not have the same educational background and many had multiple commitments in addition to school. I could not expect the same level of time commitment to learning that I had given my studies as an undergraduate in a traditional four-year college program nor that I had expected of my students in similar programs in the past.

1

And yet, in my view, these students needed more time to study than any other group I had ever worked with. I needed help and, although I received a lot of advice from colleagues, I needed a better grasp on how to help these students to be successful. I needed a "How-To" book for teaching nursing in an Associate Degree Nursing (AD) Program.

My decision to write this book derives from an intense desire to help community college students achieve success and to provide a "How-To" set of guidelines for new and not-so-new faculty teaching nursing in an Associate Degree (AD) Program. There are many books written about teaching methodology and curriculum design, but very few address the needs of the community college student. The advice and directives in these texts, which are focused on curriculum and nursing education generally, must be adapted to the needs of the AD nursing students or discarded as impractical. As women have ever-expanding career choices and as we, as a society, continue to lower expectations of high school graduates, I suspect that much of what is proposed in this book would be useful for teaching students in any generic nursing program, regardless of the institution or the educational level.

I have chosen to write a very practical and specific text, which can easily and quickly help new faculty to get a positive sense of direction as they begin their role as "teacher." Most graduate nursing school programs have, for many years, dropped their teaching track in favor of an administrative track or, more recently, a nurse practitioner track. The National League for Nurses 2000 data indicates that only 64 of the more than 375 master's programs offer a nursing education track or a post-master's certificate in teaching nursing. "Less than two percent of all full-time and part-time enrolled students are in this 'track' " (Valiga, April, 2002, paragraph 18). The rationale usually given is that graduate students were not enrolling in this teaching track because money and job availability were no longer in education but in more clinically oriented roles. This was definitely short-sighted on nursing education's part, since we no longer have a pool of potential nursing faculty with this training, and most of us with this background in teaching are approaching retirement age (Bensing, May 2000). With the current, intense nursing shortage we not only need to increase the number of nursing students, but also to provide adequately prepared faculty to teach them. Some graduate schools of nursing are now rethinking their decisions of the past and beginning to provide for a teaching major or, at least, courses in curriculum design, teaching methodology, and test construction, which would better prepare nurse educators. Berlin and Sechrist point out that "the deficiency of faculty is contributing to the general nursing shortage inasmuch as the inability to recruit and maintain adequate numbers of qualified faculty is restricting the number of students admitted to nursing programs" (Berlin & Sechrist, March/April 2002, paragraph 2). The federal government must also channel financial resources into this area of nursing to encourage more participation from colleges and universities and from future graduate students.

In addition to not participating in the more financially rewarding private and clinical sector, faculty must also deal with workload issues and the unrealistic role expectations of colleges and universities (Berlin & Sechrist, March/April 2002). A clinical lab cannot be compared to a science or language arts lab with respect to faculty time commitment, clinical expertise, or legal and ethical responsibilities. "Labs" in any nursing program deal with real people who depend on faculty to supervise students in a dramatic manner not present in other fields. The repercussions of our failure to supervise appropriately can be staggering. Our responsibility is not only to the student, but also to the clients with whom we work and the institution in which we and our students are given the opportunity to practice.

Financial remuneration for nursing faculty in state-sponsored institutions of higher education, in general, and in associate degree nursing programs, in particular, is influenced by the economic conditions of the state or commonwealth in which the institutions function. In other words, salaries and raises are more influenced by the state budget than by merit, seniority, or faculty rank. Since most associate degree faculty are focused more on teaching than on research funded by outside sources, the impact can be significant in terms of a freeze on faculty wages.

The good news is that the job market in nursing education is currently wide open at all levels. As hospitals downsize their supervisory and clinical specialist positions and as the nurse practitioner job market declines in larger cities (Berlin & Sechrist, March/April 2002) more and more masters and doctorally prepared graduates may find faculty positions in an associate degree program more appealing. Most who commit to this challenging new opportunity may not feel prepared by education or experience to take on this role and, perhaps, you may not feel you understand the needs of the nontraditional student. It is for you that this book was written.

SCOPE OF THIS BOOK

I have tried to make this book user friendly, practical, and specific. My advice is gleaned from many years of teaching to and learning from students, trial and error, workshops, research, and application. Some of the more recent works are cited in each chapter.

This text starts with an examination of associate degree nursing students and their significance to and impact on nursing. Without a good understanding of our audience, we cannot design a useful approach to helping them learn. Chapter 2 describes the rich diversity of ages, backgrounds, cultures, and educational levels that these students bring to the field. The challenge to individualize our approach in order to help these students succeed in no way diminishes the goals and objectives of a particular course or a curriculum. Graduates of community colleges pass the licensing exam at a high rate and provide excellent nurses for the community. Many go on to receive BSN and higher degrees and provide an available and quick solution for a community's nursing shortage.

Chapters 3, 4, and 5 discuss strategies specifically designed for use with community college students in small classes. Having attended a large university nursing school myself, I probably could have benefited from many of these teaching techniques used at smaller schools. However useful these tools are with any basic nursing population, they are essential if we are to retain and graduate most students in an associate degree program. Success in nursing, as in life, has less to do with age and background than it does with faculty and student attitudes and the willingness to give and receive individualized support.

Chapter 6 focuses on why some students do not make the grade and how to help them remedy the situation or at least help them to salvage their self-esteem and plan a new course of action. It is my personal belief that no educator has the right to attack or demean a student simply because the student is not performing to the teacher's expectations or does not represent what the instructor envisions as "good nursing material." However, this does not mean that we should pass everyone. It does mean that we must consider students as individuals and guide them in whatever ways seem appropriate at the time. Women's issues have an important and potentially devastating impact on the mostly female population in nursing programs and are also addressed in chapter 6. Additionally, issues involving male students are discussed in this chapter because they are implicated in the success or lack thereof for these students. Not every student who enters the nursing program will be successful; however, we must make every effort to help them with math, reading, and science skills prior to enrollment and assist them in attaining the necessary prerequisites for success in nursing. The community college was designed for and is superbly qualified to provide these services.

Chapter 7 deals with mentoring and the characteristics of an effective nursing educator at any level; these traits are particularly important for faculty in an associate degree nursing program. This is not an easy job, but hopefully it is one that gives us great satisfaction and a sense that we have made a significant impact on the lives of our students and their families. In addition, by increasing the number of new nurses, we can have an impact on the nursing shortage and the health of the communities in which we live.

The last chapter discusses the impact community college nursing programs can have on alleviating the nursing shortage. The students of these programs are often first-generation college graduates and come to us as at-risk, nontraditional students. With a little bit of help and encouragement, they can do well and many go on to get higher degrees.

ATTITUDES AND FOCUS

Most of us had a favorite teacher or mentor who greatly influenced our thinking and nursing practice. Some of us were lucky enough to have more than one. My practice as an educator was dramatically changed forever by my graduate clinical coordinator, Marianne Zalar, at the University of California at San Francisco Medical Center, School of Nursing. She introduced herself and stated that she was not our "teacher" but a "facilitator of our learning." That amazed and empowered me in an instant. I was no longer a recipient of what the "teacher" had to teach, but a co-director in the process of my growth and development as a nursing professional. It also terrified me, however, since I was now responsible for deciding what it was I wanted to learn, how I would accomplish this task, and how hard I was willing to work to make it happen. Hearing a "teacher" say this indicated to me that she was flexible, approachable, and willing to individualize the learning opportunities within the scope of her job description and the objectives of the course. As a graduate of this program, I wanted to portray this attitude and focus and become a "facilitator of learning" for others. But, not having experienced this in my own undergraduate curriculum, I wondered if it would work with generic nursing students. Trial and error and continuous reevaluation has taught me that it not only works, but it is essential to helping students progress in their own personal and professional growth. It fosters critical thinking skills, personal empowerment, and, of all things, the use of the nursing process in a real and meaningful manner. I highly recommend that you begin or continue to think of yourself as a facilitator and introduce yourself as such to your students. It may change everything!

REFERENCES

Bensing, K. (2000, May 22). Nursing Education Today, Part 2: Trends in Graduate Education. *Advance for Nurses.*

Berlin, L. E., & Sechrist, K. R. (2002, March/April). The Shortage of Doctorally Prepared Nursing Faculty: A Dire Situation. *Nursing Outlook.*

National League for Nursing (NLN). (2001, September 19). Position Statement: Lifelong Learning For Nursing Faculty. *http://www.nln.org/aboutnln/positionstate ment.htm* 10/2/02.

Valiga, T. M. (2002, April 11). The Nursing Faculty Shortage: National League for Nursing Perspective. Presentation to the National Advisory Council on Nursing Education and Practice (NACNEP). *http://www.nln.org/slides/speech.htm* 10/2/02.

2

The Associate Degree Nursing Student

Shelley F. Conroy

> *Providing an open door, community and technical colleges have become the face of the future of higher education—and of American society . . .- Community and technical colleges currently enroll 44% of all American undergraduate students and more than half of the freshmen and sophomores* (CCSSE, 2002).

Registered Nurses represent 16% of the United States' health professions. At 2.7 million in number, they are the cornerstone of the health care workforce (HRSA, 2000). One of the significant changes in the national RN population over the past 20 years has been in the proportions of the RN graduates who were prepared in the different types of educational programs (See Fig. 2.1). At 40% of the population, RNs prepared at the Associate Degree level are now the largest group of entry-level practitioners. This places the community colleges in the position of being the single largest educational institution involved in educating nurses for entry-level practice. As we struggle with the current and perhaps long-standing nursing shortage, we must do everything in our power to continue to recruit, retain, nurture, and reward this large segment of the nursing workforce.

ANALYSIS OF THE NATIONAL SURVEY SAMPLE OF REGISTERED NURSES

The data obtained in the National Survey Sample of Registered Nurses (HRSA, 2000) demonstrates that racial-ethnic minorities con-

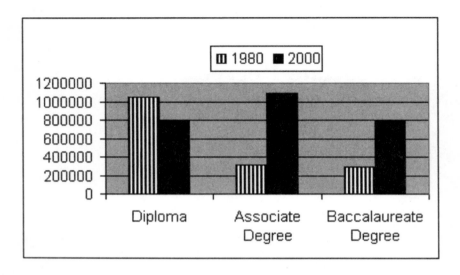

FIGURE 2.1   Distribution of RNs according to basic nursing education, 1980–2000.

United States Department of Health and Human Services Health Resources and Service Administration, Bureau of Health Professions, Division of Nursing (HRSA) (2000).

tinue to be under-represented, blacks and Hispanics being the most under-represented racial groups. Eighty-seven percent of nurses are white, while the U.S. population is reflective of 28% minorities. Additionally, only 11% of the nursing population can speak another language. When examining gender diversity in the workforce, we see that men, although their numbers have doubled in the past 20 years, comprise only 5.4% of nurses; this makes them the most significantly under-represented group in nursing.

The study data also demonstrates that younger cohorts are not replacing the aging population of nurses. In 1980, 51.3% of nurses were under age 40. In 2000, only 31.7% were less than 40 years old. The average age of all RNs is 45.2, with 40–49-year-olds being the largest age group represented in the profession. Compounding this situation are two factors: a large number of nurses start to leave the workforce at age 55, and the age of today's entry-level practitioners is increasing. The average age of the new graduate from all program types is now 30.5 years. Associate Degree graduates' average age is 33.2 years of age. This results in only approximately 22–25 years of practice for the average nursing professional and exacerbates the current nursing workforce shortage.

As a result of these findings, The Division of Nursing—Health and Human Services (HHS) is offering grants to promote workforce diversity and target young, under-represented minorities, with a focus on pre-entry preparation and retention activities. They also encourage basic nursing education to focus on projects and curricular activities that establish or expand nursing practice to increase access to primary health care in medically underserved communities, as well as educational activities to develop cultural competencies among nurses. Additional grant opportunities have been made available for programs that promote career mobility for nursing personnel (e.g., LPN to RN), flexible course scheduling, and distance learning.

IMPLICATIONS FOR ASSOCIATE DEGREE NURSING PROGRAMS

Associate degree nursing programs are ideally suited to meet the goals identified by HHS and to assist with promoting the diversity of the nursing workforce. Additionally, LPN to RN mobility programs can frequently be found in associate degree settings. The community college setting tends to be the place where one finds the highest concentration of non-traditional and ethnic minority students. Community colleges enroll 49% of all minority students in American undergraduate education (CCSSE, 2002). Because of the nature of the community college's mission, the associate degree nursing programs found there have a higher concentration of at-risk or disadvantaged learners, as well as a population with widely diverse educational backgrounds. Community colleges open their doors to all people in the community. Open access makes community colleges the gateway to economic advancement. This diversity challenges nursing educators to find the pedagogical strategies necessary to promote success and increase program retention with the special populations found in our learning environments.

ASSOCIATE DEGREE STUDENTS

The older student population is the fastest growing population in community colleges. The average age of community college students is 29. Sixty-four percent of community college students are part-time, as compared to 22% of those in four-year institutions (CCSSE, 2002). Students in these settings are three to four times more likely than those at baccalaureate institutions to possess the characteristic factors that put them at risk of not completing their degree. The fact that these students often have part-time or full-time employment, family obligations, and are frequently under-prepared for college contributes to their at-risk status. The cultural diversity found in today's community college setting also poses potential language, reading proficiency, and learning barriers for some students. There is no disputing that retention is a major dilemma facing associate degree educators today.

CHALLENGES IN THE CLASSROOM

How do these factors influence what is happening in today's classroom? The rich diversity that our students bring to the classroom challenges us to develop a portfolio of multiple pedagogical strategies for learning in order to accommodate divergent learning styles. The majority of adult learners require tactile, hands-on application opportunities. The traditional lecture method of recounting factual information is least effective with this population. The irony is that this method of instruction is most popular among today's teachers, yet the same teachers assess their students using practical application and critical thinking testing methodology. How are students supposed to acquire the critical thinking and professional judgment skills so essential for academic success, for success on the licensure examination, and for eventual success as a practitioner?

It becomes clear that faculty need to develop strategies for the classroom that help adult learners to problem-solve, think critically, and set priorities. Associate degree educators need assistance to strengthen their curricular and instructional methods in order to assure the success of their highly motivated nontraditional learners. Permit me to share with you a few examples to illustrate the challenges presented by today's students for educators in associate degree programs.

- Joanne, a veteran nursing educator in an associate degree program, teaches the first semester nursing students on a regular basis. One of her recurring teaching assignments deals with the dosage calculations unit content. On a regular basis, Joanne encounters students who need remedial assistance in how to divide, compute decimals, and convert fractions. Frequently, these students also have "math phobia." Joanne finds herself spending countless hours outside the classroom assisting these students to obtain academic support and tutoring services.

- Hank has noticed that the students who frequently have difficulty in his psychiatric nursing course are reading below the college level. When they are referred for academic support services, most are found to be reading at the sixth to eighth grade level. When Hank has the English faculty analyze his textbook they inform him that it is written at the 14th grade level.

- Sharon teaches the foundational nursing course for entering students. She meets with a new student after the first test in the course because the student has failed the exam with a significantly low score. Sharon discovers that English is this student's second language. Upon reviewing test items, it is clear that the student does not interpret the questions and answer options in the same way as students who have English as a primary language.

- Susan regularly teaches the child abuse content in her nursing program. After she teaches her class for the sophomore students, Janice comes to her office and reveals that she was sexually abused by her stepfather over a multi-year period during her adolescence. Susan spends time listening to Janice, who is still dealing with unresolved psychological issues related to her abuse. Susan assists Janice by referring her to the college's counselor and community mental health resources for abused women.

- Loretta teaches in the LPN to RN transition program at the community college. She receives a phone call from one of her students, who says she cannot make it to class for the midterm examination because her son was wounded in a drive-by shooting the previous evening.

- Jean, the nursing program director, meets with a student in her office. The student tells her that she has not been able to afford the textbook for her nursing course because her husband just left her and filed for bankruptcy. The student is contemplating withdrawal from the course so she can get a refund of her tuition to use for living expenses. The student is not eligible for financial aid at the moment because her eligibility is calculated based upon her previous year's tax return. Additionally, because it is mid-term, all grants and scholarships have already been awarded.

These are but a few examples of the life situations community college educators see on a daily basis. We all know that students must be in a state of readiness to learn in order to be successful in the classroom. There are a multitude of factors, as illustrated above, that can interfere with a student's readiness to learn, including academic prerequisite skills, emotional health, and life situations. Recruitment of gender and ethnic minority populations in order to address the diversity and workforce shortage issues in the nursing profession will also bring to the college higher numbers of disadvantaged and high-risk populations of student learners. Our challenge, then, is to develop effective teaching and mentoring strategies to promote student success and retention in associate degree nursing programs.

REFERENCES

Community College Survey of Student Engagement (CCSSE). (2002). Focusing on the face of the future. *CCSSE Highlights, Vol. 1, Issue 2.* (April, 2002).
United States Department of Health and Human Services Health Resources and Service Administration, Bureau of Health Professions, Division of Nursing (HRSA). (2000). The registered nurse population: Findings from the National Sample Survey of Registered Nurses. Washington, DC: HRSA.

3

Teaching Strategies
for the Associate Degree Student

All instruction should cultivate . . . the new student . . . systematically and rigorously by reflectively revised modes on instruction which undercut traditional student passivity and lethargy (Shaping College and University Realities, Fall, 1992, p. 26).

CHANGING PARADIGM

We and our students are being asked to do more with less. We have more students and fewer faculty. We have more students with less educational background and less available time to learn. We have shorter semesters in which to help these students learn more information than students have been asked to learn in the past. The expectations of graduates from an associate degree nursing program have recently been expanded by NLN in 2000 to include competencies in displaying appropriate professional behaviors and standards of professional practice, effective communication skills, holistic initial and ongoing assessment skills, appropriate clinical decision-making skills, appropriate caring interventions, teaching and learning skills, collaboration skills, and management skills (National League for Nursing, 2000).

What is a teacher to do? Is it possible to help today's average community college nursing student learn all she/he needs to know to pass the RN licensing exam (NCLEX-RN) and be a successful beginning practitioner in our current complex health care system? My answer to this question is a definite "yes." However, it takes dedication and creative approaches, and it mandates that we stop teaching and start listening to students and motivating and empowering them to learn. Nursing education is changing from a "sage-

13

on-the-stage" teaching paradigm, which most of us experienced in undergraduate and often graduate schools, to an interactive, student-centered learning paradigm (Fitzpatrick, July/August, 1999). The added bonus is that, as we teach our students to learn, we are modeling effective teaching strategies that they can use when teaching their patients (clients). The good news about this paradigm shift is that our students take more responsibility for their own education. The bad news is that we need to reinvent ourselves with each group of students and individualize our approach to help them become the best that they can be. So how do we do that?

First let me make it clear that teaching students at this level can be a great challenge. Instructors must be effective, practical classroom teachers as well as experienced clinical practitioners. Students at this level must feel confident that their instructor is able to care for clients and garner the respect of the staff nurses in the clinical facility. In other words, the teacher must be able to demonstrate that hands-on experience is as important as knowing what the book says. For this reason it takes more expertise to teach at this level. There is also a fine line for the instructor to walk between demonstrating his/her own clinical expertise and allowing students to develop their skills while respecting the client's right to competent care. The instructor is often in a position to make decisions in the clinical setting that require tact, diplomacy, and critical thinking with regard to the dichotomy between the student's learning needs and the client's rights. Last semester I allowed a recently homeless man to give himself an injection of insulin that the student had prepared (her first), because he firmly stated he wanted to do so. He was being discharged and my intuition was that he wanted to hang on to some semblance of his former life. I also wanted to watch his technique. The student would have another opportunity, but this client desperately needed to maintain his self-respect. The resolution to the conflict between students' needs and clients' needs may well be an area not taught in any graduate school preparation, but it is one that is developed with practice, patience, and personal sensitivity in the clinical setting. Allowing students to discuss how they felt in difficult situations and sharing your rationale for your response to a particular occurrence can teach both the student and the instructor a great deal.

TEACHING STUDENTS HOW TO LEARN

Some students need very basic help with learning how they learn best, prioritizing their time, and organizing the best method to achieve their goals. Some may even need direction in order to develop their own concrete goals. If they come from a school or work setting where someone else sets the agenda, the concept that a lot of their learning will be self-directed can be frightening to some and liberating to others.

   1.   The first thing to do is direct students to use assessment tools that help them discover their own learning style, personality profile, and/or multiple intelligence inventory and how each of these assessments directs them toward more productive ways of learning. For example, active learners learn best by doing something with the information whereas reflective learners need time to mull over the information. Visual learners need diagrams, flow-charts, videos while auditory learners need verbal discussion or reading out loud. Linear/factual learners gain insight by using specific facts in a step-by-step progression and theoretic/holistic learners like big-picture ideas and creative thinking (Katz, 2001). There are a few texts in the reference list at the end of this chapter that contain useful queries, which also can be used to assess learning styles (Ellis, 2000 and Royal, Garren, & Tutton, 2001). The questionnaires and explanations can be copied and put on reserve for students' use. Matching up the learning styles and personality of the student with several individualized strategies should help students to be more successful than if they tried to study the way everyone else does. Be sure to demonstrate that you value their expenditure of time by meeting with them collectively or separately to discuss what they discovered about themselves and how they plan to use the learning strategies suggested. These exercises can be useful anytime, but are most beneficial for students at the beginning of a semester or after they have not done well on their first test. In other words, suggest it early enough to matter. If this has been done in an orientation or study skills course, or in a previous semester, spend a few minutes at the beginning of each subsequent semester discussing their findings and how they plan to use the material this semester.

2.   Some students may need suggestions of places to study to make their time more productive. These students tend to be very practical, task-oriented adults who are easily distracted at home by the many needs of house and family, so anywhere else is usually a better place. Many students use the community college library or lab before or after class. Some prefer libraries closer to home or other locations that promote learning. This may seem like a simple decision to make, but students often come to the nursing program having done well in non-nursing courses without thinking about this variable. They have often taken only three to six credits each semester and are not ready for the workload of a 7- to 10-credit nursing course, which includes lab (clinical) hours.

3.   Community college students may or may not be very educationally sophisticated, so nothing should be assumed. Advice about pre-reading activities such as getting organized, activating prior knowledge about topics, previewing text and chapter, asking questions, and using questions at the end of the chapter (Faulkner & Stahl, 1999) may need to be taught and/or encouraged. I have taught a "test taking skills in nursing" course for many years (see Box 5.4 for essential elements of this course) and am continually amazed at how some of the simplest suggestions can profoundly influence students' progress. Even suggesting that an increased amount of time is needed to comprehend a nursing text, with its new vocabulary and higher reading level, is helpful. Some students may continue to use strategies that have proven successful in non-nursing courses but not in nursing courses simply because they do not know of others to try.

4.   The students who are having difficulty may also need help in becoming more active readers and in using the many charts, graphs, care plans, and "in a nutshell" boxes that the textbook may use to analyze and synthesize the material. Many students skip this content without realizing its value. Students should be encouraged often to look up new words and write the definition in the text margin, along with their own familiar interpretation. Annotations, outlines, mind mapping, and pictures that reinforce details have become a lost art for students who do not think they have time for these strategies. Teaching students to number a list of signs and symptoms or prioritized nursing interventions in the book margins is more effective than highlighting this list. Drawing circles and arrows that connect information, as in mind mapping, is a very visual means of demonstra-

ting relationships. Using a different color for the *first* or *most important* point to remember is also helpful to many students as they read information. For a very visual learner, the technique of developing a movie in his or her head of client scenarios unfolding as the chapter is read is also an active reading strategy that increases retention of content. This, however, requires some clinical experience for effective use. Students who have had several clinicals could visualize themselves transferring a client from the bed to a wheelchair using the correct body mechanics. Likewise, they could "see" a client who demonstrated a particular set of signs and symptoms and then take appropriate action in there mind's eye. Interactive video discs are also helpful at teaching students the consequences of their actions or inactions and should be used at all levels to teach appropriate nursing interventions. For the auditory learner, reading outloud, perhaps even into a tape recorder, improves alertness and concentration. Students who have a long commute to school can listen to the tape in the car to increase comprehension. While outlining or mind mapping, a student could use arrows to help with concepts of cause and effect; numbers can be used to indicate a list of signs and symptoms or interventions, as well as to prioritize this list. These strategies cause the student to interact with the material while reading, so that information and concepts are pushed into long-term memory. In the long run, this shortens future study time (Falkner & Stahl, 1999).

TAKING RATIONALE TO THE CELLULAR LEVEL

As a learning facilitator, you can help students to focus on rationale for interventions by getting scientific. Simplistic explanations are only short-term solutions. In order to help the student apply scientific principles and concepts to new problems, these principles must be learned well in biology, chemistry, anatomy and physiology. Students often must be helped to remember or relearn these basics before focusing on their nursing application. In order to keep this depth of understanding alive, every subsequent class should be taught in such a way that concepts of asepsis, fluid, electrolyte, and acid-base balance; actions of the sympathetic and para-sympathetic nervous system; as well as the basic functions of all the body systems should be reinforced as they pertain to new topics in medical-surgical nursing and the nursing specialties. This, of course, is easier said than done.

If your plan is to reinforce basic concepts, you must have them fresh in *your* mind. Some of us had great science courses and possess a font of scientific knowledge from which to draw. Those of us who do not, however, can review current science textbooks that students have used in prior courses and refer them to specific pages or chapters. I have often asked students to "read it again for the first time." Now that they need to know the information in order to understand the nursing care of a client, it will make more sense to them and they will be more likely to remember it. Or you could attend some of the science classes the students are taking or take an advanced physiology course yourself. Teaching nursing at the associate degree level is not for the faint of heart.

I have had the privilege (although I did not think so at the time) of teaching in each of the first three semesters of a four-semester nursing program. Since my specialty, maternal-newborn nursing, is placed in the third semester, I can make reference to what the students learned in fundamentals of nursing and beginning medical-surgical nursing courses and help them to apply this material to relevant aspects of my course. I do this by asking them to recall normal adult values for vital signs, blood sugar, bladder capacity, or urine output in ccs per kilogram of body weight. Then I compare these values to the changes that occur during pregnancy and postpartum, giving rationale for these physiologic changes. I then build on this to help the students understand pathophysiologic states such as pregnancy-induced hypertension or postpartum hemorrhage. Not only does this method engage the students in a discussion of previously learned material, it also gives greater significance to the new material and helps them remember all of it. So what happens if no one remembers the answers to my questions? If I can not tease it out of them with a few clinical examples, then I ask them to find the answer for the next class or clinical, or to e-mail it to me. This usually only happens once. The students then usually review related material prior to or during their reading for each subsequent class and come prepared to participate. Not only does this make the class more interesting, it also teaches students how to read their textbook more actively and begin to put the pieces together themselves. If students are in small classes, this approach makes keeping track of and assessing student effort and thinking skills more manageable.

If classes are large (greater than 20) this approach can also be used during clinical conference discussions, since each clinical instructor usually only supervises eight to twelve students at one time. Students who do not prepare for class or clinical in this fashion rarely do well on tests. This fact should be pointed out to them as part of your guidance for success. Preparation for clinical should also be part of the student's clinical evaluation. Anything and everything should be used, as necessary, to induce students to study in a manner that is most likely to increase their learning and their success in nursing school and in the profession.

I also teach cardiac assessment in a health assessment course to first semester students; I always start the class by asking students to trace a drop of blood through the heart and lungs from the inferior vena cava to the aorta. They do this in writing and turn it in for my feedback. Students are told that they can use a drawing, words, arrows to indicate flow, or any other method they choose. This material, of course, is reviewed in the first few pages of the assigned chapter. A student may not have read the chapter, but still know the information, which is to be celebrated. However, whether or not students have read the chapter, they often reverse the right and left side of the heart and put the trip through the lungs in most unproductive places. I can then use this feedback to point out that memorizing is a very short term solution to learning and should be replaced by an understanding of physiology and the "whys" of bodily function. If students have read the material and are still unable to be accurate, I point out that they are not reading actively for the significance of the material. They must begin to ask themselves questions while reading, draw pictures and arrows, point to areas on their own body, or use their fingers to make the pictures in the text come alive and make a mental imprint.

The follow up to this health assessment exercise is a question to second semester students, which explores their understanding of the rationale for why a piece of a deep vein thrombosis can only lodge in the lungs, causing a pulmonary embolism. As a further explanation of the circulatory system in third-semester maternity and nursing of children courses, questions about the complexities of fetal circulation, why and how fetal structures close at birth, and the congenital cardiac anomalies that arise if they do not are easier to teach and learn. By using a method of teaching that connects current content to past learning, we also teach the student the usefulness of doing this on his/her own, while reading for each of the next classes of the course and in the future. Although it increases class and clinical preparation time for the student, it decreases study time for tests and for the final exams. It also usually translates into better grades and more clinical self-confidence. Table 3.1 gives additional examples of the use of basic concepts throughout the curriculum.

Clinical papers are another way of pushing students to get to the cellular level. In-depth scientific rationale for nursing interventions should be required. Sources should include anatomy and physiology texts, health assessment texts, fundamentals of nursing texts, and current relevant journal articles as well as the current course textbook. Care plan books, although helpful in organizing thoughts on appropriate nursing care, are less useful in an exploration of concrete physiology and pathophysiology to explain why or how interventions work for this particular client problem. Understanding the science behind nursing interventions will increase the student's ability to remember content, prioritize interventions, and function clinically. Memorizing a laundry list of actions will not.

STORYTELLING TO ENHANCE LEARNING

Storytelling can be used in multiple ways to accomplish several purposes. Banks-Wallace, in her article on the use of storytelling to provide holistic care to women, lists the following purposes:

1. to gather pertinent client information
2. to strengthen client-nurse communication
3. to provide client education
4. to enhance staff and clinical development

She points out that relevant stories shared between practitioner and client and among clients break down barriers, create a connection, and express cultural values that might not otherwise be assessed (Banks-Wallace, 1999, January/February, p. 20).

Nontraditional students often have many personal examples related to class discussions. If the student is a licensed practical nurse (LPN) or a certified nursing assistant (CNA), personal clinical examples can be added to the mix of ideas and images that a student

TABLE 3.1 Scientific Rationale Across the Curriculum

Concepts	Fundamentals of Nursing Health Assessment	Medical-Surgical Nursing	Maternity Nursing	Nursing of Children	Psychiatric/Mental Health Nursing
Acid-Base Balance	Respiratory & metabolic balances/ Imbalances	Diabetes/ respiratory causes CNS depressant overdose General anesthesia	L & D— hyperventilation Diabetes in pregnancy	Diabetes in children Asthma	Anxiety disorders
Circulation	Auscultation of heart/heart sounds Circulation & oxygenation basics	Cardiac/ respiratory problems Venous & arterial clots DVT/pulmonary embolism Use of anticoagulants Hyperlipidemia Hemorrhage, shock, strokes	Fetal circulation → NB Placental circulation Placental abruption Postpartum hemorrhage	Cardiac anomalies Necrotizing enterocolitis Intracranial hemorrhage	Dementia Hematologic disorders caused by medications

(continued)

TABLE 3.1 (continued)

Concepts	Fundamentals of Nursing Health Assessment	Medical-Surgical Nursing	Maternity Nursing	Nursing of Children	Psychiatric/Mental Health Nursing
Electrolyte Balance	Effects of vomiting/diarrhea S/S of hypo & hyper	GI problems in adults	L & D—hyperventilation	GI problems in children	Eating disorders
Fight or Flight Mechanisms	Sympathetic & parasympathetic responses Effects on V. S., output Levels of anxiety	Effects on V. S., Circulation, Respiratory, GI & renal disorders Medications used to control effects of fight or flight	Effects on AP, L & D, PP & NB Effects on teaching/learning Violence/abuse during pregnancy	Effects on children Appropriate treatment Effects on g & d, fears, etc. Child abuse	Catatonia Anxiety/panic disorders Depression Violence/abuse of the elderly
Fluid Balance	Oncotic pressure/edema Hydrostatic pressure BP & pulse	Liver & Renal disease Dehydration in elderly	Antepartal dehydration Hyperemesis Gravidarum Fluid balance in newborn Pregnancy induced hypertension	Effects of dehydration in small children	Psychogenic overhydration Fluid & electrolyte balance related to medications

TABLE 3.1 (continued)

Concepts	Fundamentals of Nursing Health Assessment	Medical-Surgical Nursing	Maternity Nursing	Nursing of Children	Psychiatric/ Mental Health Nursing
Infection Control	Chain of infection Standard precautions Disease-specific precautions	Communicable diseases MRSA/VRS Wound infection Immuno-compromized client	Standard Precautions in L&D, postpartum & nursery NB s/s of infection Care of the immuno-compromised NB or premature infant HIV transmission to fetus	Immunization schedule Immuno-compromized children	Effects of depression & mental illness on immuno-competence
Nutrition	Food pyramid Functions of proteins, fats, carbohydrates, water, vitamins, and minerals	Diets for various disorders	Diets during pregnancy, breastfeeding, postoperative cesarean delivery	Diet - infancy - toddler/ preschool age - school age - adolescence	Obesity Eating disorders

(continued)

TABLE 3.1 *(continued)*

Concepts	Fundamentals of Nursing Health Assessment	Medical-Surgical Nursing	Maternity Nursing	Nursing of Children	Psychiatric/ Mental Health Nursing
Pain	Physiology of pain Pain fibers & large fibers Function of nervous system Routes of meds; onset	Pain control: acute/chronic Drugs & equigesic dosing General anesthesia Non-pharmacologic pain relief	Gate block theory used in L & D & Postpartum Local & regional anesthesia/ analgesia	Pain response in children Useful pain relief options in children	Phantom pain Malingering Pain disorders Somatic disorders
Valsalva Maneuvers	Basic Bowel Elimination Effects on Cardiac & Respiratory systems	Effects on cardiac and respiratory diseases	L & D—Pushing	Cardiac & Respiratory effects	Breath holding

already has. These "stories" may or may not help the student to remember content, to put it in proper perspective, or to think critically about the nurse's role in the prevention and care of clients affected. It all depends on the validity of the context of the student's experiences. If students are not allowed and encouraged to express these thoughts of prior experiences, the context in which they view new data will never be appreciated. Students, as well as the public at large, build on prior knowledge. That is how we all learn and grow. If the prior knowledge is on target and typical of whatever concept or disease entity is discussed, then it is a very useful part of learning. If, however, their story or experience is atypical or erroneously remembered, then it will confuse and/or mislead the student. Have you ever wondered why students answer questions in such a bizarre manner? It may be that, despite what was said in class or stated in the text, their personal experiences and/or cultural biases superceded the content and led them to choose the wrong answer. We must allow students to voice these experiences as part of a discussion of the topic so that we can assess for misinformation and atypical experiences in order to clarify and reinterpret the facts students need to remember.

Before students will share personal stories and experiences, they must trust the instructor and their classmates to respect them and their confidences. At the beginning of the semester and/or during a particular class, "the rules" for such sharing should be laid out. Everything that is shared in class is for the purpose of enhanced learning. It should not leave the classroom. Tape recording of such stories should not be allowed. In fact, the nursing program in which I teach restricts the use of tape recorders; only those students with documented learning disabilities may use a tape recorder if it has been prescribed. Taping a lecture is a poor substitute for coming prepared to class and having an outline of the class content prepared. Routine use of tape recorders in nursing classes by the majority of students poses a legal and ethical dilemma in that it invariably breaches patient or personal confidentiality. Who else is listening to the tapes? Family members and nonnursing friends may recognize or think they recognize the person described.

Next, the faculty should share stories and examples that illustrate the concepts being discussed. Personal and clinical excerpts as well as students' examples can be used. Faculty should have obtained verbal permission from previous students for such use in case students in subsequent classes recognize the particulars of the story and realize to whom they belong. Details should be minimized and school policy should be followed. Enhanced communication between faculty and students, fostered by the use of "shared experiences," makes students more willing to expose potential vulnerabilities and cultural uniqueness to illustrate the concept more clearly or to discuss the variations and differences that a story represents. Demonstrate sensitivity to the student's feelings when he or she gives an example that is not on track and guide the student back to the material and concepts that must be remembered. There are probably others in the class who have headed down a similar path, leading to inaccurate information, a wrong answer on a test, and, more importantly, inappropriate nursing interventions in a clinical setting.

Stories used by instructors do not have to be factual or real. They can be constructed to fit the point being made. Faculty can also create client scenarios and have students fill in the pieces. These I call my "what if" scenarios. After providing some client data, I might ask if there are any pieces missing that should be gathered before a plan of care is constructed. "What if" a plan is based on the data presented, what care might be missed or given erroneously? "What if" an added piece of information happened next, would you change the care plan and, if so, in what way? As you can see, storytelling can teach not only concepts and nursing interventions, but also critical thinking skills.

Since storytelling can be time consuming, it should be used judiciously. Clinical discussion might lend itself better to exploration of personal and clinical examples. However, if all clinical groups are to benefit, communication between the classroom teacher and each clinical instructor is mandatory. Concepts that might be best taught in small clinical group discussions during a post conference include legal and ethical issues, values, confidentiality, professional behavior, client and family rights, and cultural considerations. We might also include discussions about what it means to be nonjudgmental and how our nursing care is influenced by our attitudes about such topics as drug addiction, smoking, alcoholism, abortion, homosexuality, and sexually transmitted diseases, including AIDS and other communicable diseases. This is certainly not an exhaustive list, but these discussions should be part of every course, in order to prepare future nurses to act professionally, holistically, ethically, and legally in caring for their present and future clients. Table 4.1 in the next chapter outlines how these concepts can be carried across the curriculum.

HUMOR IN THE CLASSROOM

In order to use humor in the classroom, an educator has to possess a degree of self-confidence and humility. After all, what you think is funny may not be so perceived by students. This may depend on how clinically savvy they are or how up-tight they are about their studies or the subject matter discussed. Community college students, in my opinion, are much more appreciative of the use of humor in the classroom than are younger or more intensely serious, "education for education's sake" students in university settings. Our nontraditional learners have a wealth of life experiences that can form the basis of camaraderie between teacher and student. However, the caveat remains that humor should be focused on enhancing learning and not, in itself, the point. It is also never okay to make students or patients, in general, or any one particular person the basis for laughter. Humor should not be confused with cleverness or sarcasm. Instructors who use humor must also avoid hidden agendas. All of the above could destroy the sense of trust and connection that an educator should be trying to develop between herself/himself and the students.

Humor creates a positive learning situation, often improves problem solving, and promotes an exchange of ideas (Lowenstein & Bradshaw, 2001). If you have never thought of yourself as funny, try to form a mental picture of the concept you are trying to teach. Turn it around, inside out, or backward and see if you find it funny. Then use it with students to demonstrate the absurdity of understanding the concept that way. You may or may not get a laugh, but you will make your point. For example, you can put an erroneous charting entry on an overhead to illustrate the need for accuracy and logical sequencing in charting. There are many of them in the humor corner of nursing journals and there are even some on the internet. You can also tell pertinent stories of your own personal and/or clinical experiences. Using overheads with an enlarged, relevant comic strip or a drawing from a study skills text, or a book on nursing humor, such as the ones in Fran London's *Whinorrhea and Other Nursing Diagnoses* (1995), is less personally anxiety provoking. My personal favorite cartoons include "Ziggy," "Sally Forth," "For Better or for Worst," "Zits," "Fox Trot," and "Rose is Rose." In fact, I start each day reading the comics to set a positive mood and look for cartoons that I can use, often that day, or in the future. Have no fear; the use of humor can be learned. It is a skill after all, and all skills can be learned. Have we not told our students this enough times to believe it ourselves? And if your attempt at humor falls flat, remember that timing is everything. Try it again later in the semester, when students have a better perspective on who you are and whether or not they can trust you. Or try humor again with a different group of students. Just like anything else, what works with some does not always work with others.

TECHNOLOGY IN NURSING EDUCATION

The future of any field of study today involves the emerging technologies. We must incorporate technology into nursing education as a strategy that increases student involvement in the learning process. Because community college students tend to be older and less affluent than those attending four-year institutions, and because the mission statement of most community colleges involves access to education, we cannot mandate that each student have a personal computer or be able to access the internet from home. We must, however, provide staffed computer labs and mandate a basic computer course as part of our curriculum. This does not mean that our students will all be computer savvy when they take clinical nursing courses. But it does mean that we can require at least some of their paperwork to be computer-generated, and that the Internet be used as a research tool. We can use such course management systems as BlackBoard or Web CT to provide students access to syllabi, notes, and assignments. Since some students may only be able to access this material at the college, all announcements must be posted in advance to allow for timely access by all students. When we assign a web search, we must be prepared to offer a lot of guidance about where to look and how to proceed, as well as actual hands on and sometimes hand-holding directions in campus computer labs. A lab assistant might do this, but it may also need to be done by educators, whether or not we are fortunate enough to have a lab assistant. Some of us are recent converts to technology and can empathize with our older students' struggles. We cannot dismiss them as incompetent. When we add a helping hand and deserved respect for prior accomplishments to students' intense desire to learn, who knows what they can accomplish?

As we use technology in our courses, we need to remember that enhanced quality and quantity of communication between faculty and students is what is really important. "In a student-faculty survey at Wake Forest University in Winston Salem, NC, for example, 87% of respondents attributed increased learning to better communication. By contrast, only 20% gave credit to the increased quality of classroom presentations (for example, with PowerPoint)" (Brown, November, 2000, p. 28). This author went on to list ways that communication can be enhanced by technology, such as providing the e-mail addresses of faculty and students who have e-mail and encouraging electronic correspondence for individual or group responses or communication between students. Another way is the timely use of announcements and reminders on blackboard or other course management systems, as already discussed.

As technology continues to invade every aspect of our lives, more and more students will have experience and personal equipment to add to their strategies for learning. As we develop web-based courses and move toward distance education and away from the classroom, it will become more and more difficult to individualize our approach to facilitating learning. Clinical courses will always have a lab component, but it may not be under our direct supervision (for example: use of preceptors' and virtual clinicals). Telecommunication technology provides on-demand, flexible learning solutions that will impact our future students and enable them to continue their educational pursuits without regard to time and space (von Holzen, November, 2000). It will empower them to become perpetual learners in classrooms without boundaries. If my snail mail does not deceive me, nursing in the four-year and graduate programs is progressing rapidly in this direction. It behooves educators in associate degree programs to prepare students to take their rightful place in this education revolution.

SURVEY OF TEACHING STRATEGIES

As part of my preparation to write this book, I distributed a survey that listed teaching strategies to a group of faculty at the Fall 2001 meeting of the Virginia Counsel of Associate Degree Nursing Educators (VaCADNE). My purpose was fourfold:

1. to assess which strategies were used most and least frequently by faculty experienced in teaching associate degree nursing students;

2. to see if strategies changed based on whether the students were in the first or the second year of the program;
3. to get more suggested strategies to add to this list; and
4. to encourage educators to think about their methodology and perhaps add new strategies that they had not thought about using.

I used a 4-point scale to avoid answers that could be classified as "middle of the road." I wanted to see a clear-cut distinction between strategies used often or routinely and those rarely or never used. The final list of teaching strategies is found in Box 3.1 and could be used periodically with new and seasoned teachers to enhance discussions of how best to increase the success rate of the student population that we serve. I encourage others to add to and refine this list to meet their own needs.

Not surprisingly, I found that the strategies of providing extra study sessions and helping students to evaluate their own learning style were used more often with first year students, while the use of seminars and assigned in-class presentations by students were strategies more often used with second year students. I was, however, puzzled by the minimal use of practice test questions, test questions in the text or on CDs accompanying the text, and quizzes prior to a test. It is my belief that students, especially nontraditional students, need experience answering higher level nursing test questions. This experience should not come at the expense of their grades, even in the first semester.

My other discovery was that the strategies used by educators who taught both first- and second-year students varied little, if at all, for both groups. It seems to me that once we have socialized students to "think like a nurse," we need to treat them differently and expect more knowledge, ability, and critical thinking skills in their last two semesters than we did in their first two. My only conclusion is that faculty expectations of first-year students may be too high or, more likely, those of second year students too low. All faculty who teach across the curriculum should be aware of the strategies they use and evaluate the appropriateness and effectiveness of these strategies for each level of student. Many of the strategies listed in the survey in Box 3.1 are discussed in this chapter as well as Chapters 4, 5, and 6.

BOX 3.1 Faculty Survey of Teaching Strategies Used in Associate Degree Nursing Programs

Please rate according to the following scale and differentiate between 1st and 2nd year

1 never use   2 sometimes use   3 often use   4 routinely use

Teaching strategies that I have found to be effective in helping students who are having difficulty in the nursing program include:

		1st year	2nd year
1.	Providing class notes	____	____
2.	Providing practice test questions	____	____
3.	Referring them to test questions in text, etc.	____	____
4.	Providing extra study sessions	____	____
5.	Providing individualized help	____	____
6.	Use of demonstration to make a point	____	____
7.	Use of non-nursing examples in class	____	____
8.	Use of clinical examples in class	____	____
9.	Relating new concepts to concepts previously learned	____	____
10.	Use of discussion in the classroom	____	____
11.	Use of role play in the classroom	____	____
12.	Assigning students to present material	____	____
13.	Assigning students to present concept mapping of content to be covered	____	____
14.	Assigning topics for research	____	____
15.	Providing study guide handouts	____	____
16.	Providing clinical guides to aide in applying new classroom material to clinical setting	____	____
17.	Use of humor to make a point in class	____	____
18.	Being passionate about the subject	____	____
19.	Use of case studies to teach critical thinking	____	____
20.	Use of seminars to reinforce learning	____	____
21.	Use of computer-assisted instruction (CAI)	____	____
22.	Use of quizzes prior to tests	____	____
23.	Use of students' prior experience to explain content	____	____
24.	Helping students to evaluate their learning style	____	____
25.	Changing method of presentation based on learning needs of each student group	____	____
26.	Varying presentation methods within a class period to include lecture, video, computer application, discussion, etc.	____	____
27.	Provide nursing tutors from prior class	____	____
28.	Encourage the organization of study groups	____	____

Please add any other strategies that you have used to overcome student difficulties. In which year were they used? How effective were they for the individual or group of students?

REFERENCES

Banks-Wallace, J. (1999, January/February). Storytelling as a Tool for Providing Holistic Care to Women. *MCN*, p. 20.

Brown, D. G. (2000, November). The Low Hanging Fruit. *Syllabus*, p. 28.

Ellis, D. (2000). *Becoming a Master Student* (9th ed.). Boston: Houghton Mifflin Company.

Faulkner, A., & Stahl, D. (1999). *Reading Strategies for Nursing and Allied Health*. Boston: Houghton in Nursing (3rd ed.). Gaithersburg, MD: Aspen Publishers, Inc.

National League for Nursing (NLN). (2000). *National League for Nursing's Educational Competencies for Graduates of Associate Degree Nursing Programs*. Boston: Jones and Bartlett Publishers.

Royall, C. D., Garren, C. M., & Tutton, R. J. (2001). *Your Journey Begins Here . . . JTCC: Your Path to Success*. Dubuque, IA: Kendall Hunt Publishing Company.

Shaping College and University Realities. (1992, Fall). *Critical Thinking: Shaping the Mind of the 21st Century*. p. 26.

von Holzen, R. (2000, November). A Look at the Future of Higher Education. *Syllabus*. pp. 57 & 65.

Mifflin Company.

Fitzpatrick, J. J. (1999, July/August). Steps on a Journey from Learning to Teaching. *Nursing and Health Care Perspectives,* p. 179.

Katz, J. R. with Carter, C., Bishop, J. & Kravits, S. L. (2001). *Keys to Nursing Success*. Upper Saddle River, NJ: Prentice Hall.

London, F. (Ed.). (1995). *Whinorrhea and Other Nursing Diagnoses*. Mesa, AZ: Journal of Nursing Jocularity Publishing, Inc.

Lowenstein, A. J., & Bradshaw, M. J. (2001). *Fuszard's Innovative Teaching Strategies*

4

Socialization into the Nursing Profession

Identifying learning outcomes is essential in ensuring that the emerging student is fit to practice. The question of how a nurse becomes socialized into the nursing profession remains of critical importance (Howkins & Ewens, 1999, p. 41).

SOCIALIZATION AS A PROCESS

Socialization into any profession cannot be accomplished in a lecture format. Values, ethics, and legal issues must be discussed with many "what ifs" and "for instances" and "if this, then whats." Presenting concepts such as the American Nurse Association Code of Ethics or Principles and Practices of Nursing is just a beginning. Each point must be explained using several examples. Generating discussion about what students think of these principles and how they see themselves applying principles in a real world setting helps to change thinking and thus behaviors. Some may have no difficulty with all or most principles, while others may wonder what they have gotten themselves into. The Code of Ethics is found at the beginning of most Fundamentals of Nursing texts and is usually discussed early in the first semester, along with legal issues and nonjudgmental caring behavior. It is often not brought up again in the curriculum unless there is a clinical occurrence or a current event reported in the newspaper that causes concern over ethics or legal behavior. If we want to move students through the process of acculturation into nursing, we first of all have to allow for the process to occur, and then encourage its progression over time by bringing it up in a variety of different contexts, in ever expanding examples throughout the curriculum. Table 4.1 suggests several examples of how this can

TABLE 4.1 Professionalism Concepts Across the Curriculum

Concepts	Nursing Fundamentals; Health Assessment	Medical-Surgical Nursing	Maternity Nursing	Nursing of Children	Psych/Mental Health Nursing
Communication	• Nurse-client relationship • Interview skills • Health history • Therapeutic techniques • Documentation • Non-therapeutic communication • Non-verbal communication • Attending skills • Charting skills • Reporting skills	• Health history • Communication project • Teaching/learning principles • Documentation • End-of-shift report	• Antepartum, labor & delivery, postpartum health history • Teaching/learning principles in antepartal, intrapartal, postpartal, and newborn care	• Communication using knowledge of growth and development • Teaching/learning principles used with children of various ages • Teaching parents	• Interpersonal process recordings • Therapeutic communication with clients with various mental illnesses in a variety of settings

TABLE 4.1 *(continued)*

Concepts	Nursing Fundamentals; Health Assessment	Medical-Surgical Nursing	Maternity Nursing	Nursing of Children	Psych/Mental Health Nursing
Legal Issues	• Sources of law • Standards of care • Good Samaritan laws • Licensure • Informed consent • Advance directives • Controlled substances • Student nurse liability • Prescriptive authority • Incident reports • Use of restraints • Chain of command	• Organ & tissue donation • HIV • Fall risks • Medication errors • Safety • ER, ICU care standards • OR, anesthesia care standards • Care of inmates in a hospital setting • Abandonment • Short-staffing • Mandatory over-time	• Abortion laws • Birth control • Use & interpretation of fetal monitors in pregnancy & labor • Assessment of complications in antepartal, intrapartal, postpartal, and newborn care	• Safety & supervision of children of varying ages • Supervision of care given by child's parents • Medication safety & pediatric dosage calculations	• Voluntary commitment • Involuntary commitment • Use of restraints • Suicide • Duty to warn • Confidentiality

(continued)

TABLE 4.1 *(continued)*

Concepts	Nursing Fundamentals; Health Assessment	Medical-Surgical Nursing	Maternity Nursing	Nursing of Children	Psych/Mental Health Nursing
Ethical Issues	• Client's Rights and Responsibilities • Client-centered care • Health care ethics • Steps in an Ethical dilemma • Cultural and religious sensitivity	• Actual ethical dilemmas • Managed care • Client's refusal of care • Signing out against medical advise (AMA) • End-of-life issues	• In-vitro fertilization • Saving very premature infants • Biomedical research • Access to care • Use of fetal tissue • Gene and stem cell therapy • Fetal therapy	• Cessation of treatment for child • Refusal to stop treatment • Court ordered treatment	• Boundaries • Transference • Countertransference • Confidentiality vs. mandatory reporting

TABLE 4.1 (*continued*)

Concepts	Nursing Fundamentals; Health Assessment	Medical-Surgical Nursing	Maternity Nursing	Nursing of Children	Psych/Mental Health Nursing
Nonjudgmental Attitude	• The Basics • Elderly • Unwashed • Mutilated • Criminals • Minority groups • Sexual orientation	• HIV • Homosexuality • Homelessness • Poverty • Non-compliance • Morbid obesity	• Violence and abuse during pregnancy • Adolescent pregnancy • Rape • Abortion • Yelling in labor • Unwed mothers	• Child abuse • Poor parenting • Violent behavior in children • Pedophilia	• Anti-social behavior • Non-compliance with meds • Sociopaths • Malingerers • Homelessness • Alternative life styles • Elder abuse • Somatic complaints

(continued)

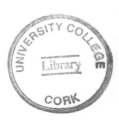

TABLE 4.1 (*continued*)

Concepts	Nursing Fundamentals; Health Assessment	Medical-Surgical Nursing	Maternity Nursing	Nursing of Children	Psych/Mental Health Nursing
Values	• Values Clarification • Personal Values • Cultural Values • Religious Values	• Use of alcohol • Smoking cessation • Avoidance of drug abuse • Following MD orders	• Prenatal care • Avoidance of drugs, smoking, alcohol in pregnancy • Birth control • Client's refusal of pain meds, epidural, blood	• Parental refusal of meds and treatment for minors • Parental refusal of blood transfusions for minors	• Drug abuse • Alcohol abuse • Fear of Muslims after 9/11 • Beliefs about mental illness & psychotherapy

be accomplished. Communication is a difficult concept to understand and communication skills are a lifetime effort. We could start with "interviewing techniques" in either the fundamentals of nursing course or in health assessment, depending on its placement in the curriculum. Practicing with a lab partner the interviewing skills necessary to gather a health history is a useful exercise for beginning students. I ask students to share their reaction to the manner in which questions were asked of them and the nonverbals which accompanied them. Students learn from each other how it feels to be interviewed and develop more insightful ways of gathering information.

Students use communication skills in a variety of ways during their first semester. They usually complete an assessment form on their client, practice narrative and computerized charting, and begin to report off to the instructor and to the staff nurse after a clinical assignment is completed. Medical-surgical nursing students often complete several client assessments, as well as a communication project. They often learn teaching and learning principles, which help them to move further into client teaching. For maternity and nursing of children students, great emphasis is placed on client and family teaching, while psychiatric nursing students concentrate mostly on the art of communication with mental health clients and their families and in groups. Communication skills are increasingly needed to obtain an adequate client history, to record it accurately, and to report it in a comprehensive and meaningful manner. The emphasis in each semester is the improvement of communication skills verbally, in writing, and through the electronic media. My list of other concepts important to the socialization of students into nursing is, by no means, all-inclusive.

It is important to keep in mind that behavior changes over time and that generic students are, by definition, not already health professionals. If we want to have an open dialogue with students about their fundamental beliefs, *we* have to be nonjudgmental and caring. We have to allow them to grow and adapt to the rigors of the nursing profession. We cannot penalize them for dissenting views or attitudes as they begin the process of learning what nursing is all about. We can, however, hold them accountable for knowing the facts of the profession of nursing, as taught in class and stated in the textbooks. Attitude and behavior changes can come later and must at least be assessed clinically in each nursing course. Marton, Dall'Alba, and

Beaty (1993) describe this internalization of learning in their report on the six conceptions of learning. They list, in order, reasons for learning: (1) to increase one's knowledge, (2) to reproduce this knowledge on tests, (3) to apply knowledge to specific circumstances, (4) to increase one's understanding of the broader meaning of something, (5) to see concepts in new and different ways, and (6) to learn so as to change as a person (Martin, Dall'alba, & Beaty, 1993).

CARING AND BEING NONJUDGMENTAL

The ethic of caring is another nursing value that must be developed and nurtured in students. Most of our students, thankfully, come to us with altruistic aspirations. However, we must help them to individualize and elevate their desire to help others to a more professional level. In other words, we need to help them to use empathy rather than sympathy; to teach the client how to do as much for himself as his condition will allow, rather than doing everything for him. We teach this best by the example of how we treat students. I have heard colleagues recount stories of educators in their undergraduate and graduate programs who stated at the beginning of a course that no one ever made it easy for them and they were not about to make it easy for the students in their class. Why do we persist in "killing our young?" This attitude, in my opinion, has no place in *any* nursing curriculum, and certainly not in an Associate Degree program. If we are to graduate students who are caring and respectful professionals, we must, as faculty, care for and respect students. These are adults with varied life experiences, which may have helped or hindered their progress thus far in the often daunting task of getting into the nursing program. They have often overcome many obstacles, such as poor educational preparation, financial difficulties, and family and work constraints to make it to our classrooms. We owe them the respect that such a struggle alone should garner. It is easy to accept students who are similar to oneself. It is quite another thing to welcome into our ranks someone who looks and acts differently, who comes from a different background, ethic group, or culture, and whose prior experiences may threaten our sense of "who would make a good nurse." Being nonjudgmental really is tough when *we* have to demonstrate this quality to *all* of our students.

A survey of 8,000 New England nurses done by researchers Joan Riley and Sara Fry in 2000 reported that the most frequent ethical conflicts involved protecting patients' rights and human dignity, and respecting/not respecting informed consent to treatment (Riley & Fry, May 2000). Obviously, having the beginning students learn the American Hospital Association's *Patients' Bill of Rights and Responsibilities* is a given. We must also use past and present examples of nurses who understand its meaning and demonstrate it by supporting and advocating for the client and family. This is especially difficult when a client's decisions go against medical advice or differ from what the student would do under similar circumstances. We can teach a systematic approach such as the very practical one advocated by Stabinski, which includes the following components: indications and desired outcomes of treatment; client/family views of treatment based on their values, and cultural and religious beliefs; quality of life issues and their meaning to the client and to everyone discussing the dilemma; financial and other boundaries that pertain to the dilemma (Stabinski, May, 2000). The client and family must live with whatever decision is made, and so their informed input is paramount. Students must be helped to understand this by participating in pertinent discussion of ethical issues throughout the curriculum (see examples in Table 4.1). Observing an ethics committee meeting at a local hospital during their last semester could be a valuable culminating experience in this area.

We can deal with legal issues in a similar fashion, by teaching the facts of the law with regard to nursing and the difference between a tort or intentional act and unintentional negligence. Each semester should have specific objectives related to legal issues relevant to the area of nursing studied. Table 4.1 has some examples. Other examples that are of local interest or have been in the news also ought to be discussed so that students can learn to make informed decisions using facts and current law. Observing the discussion of a malpractice or drug diversion case at the state board of nursing would be an invaluable experience for students in their last semester of a nursing program. If this is not feasible, at least a discussion of the published notes and disposition of such a case would greatly enhance a student's awareness and understanding of the ramifications of laws as they apply to the nursing profession.

CLIENT ADVOCACY

In order to help students see themselves as client advocates, we need to help them increase their assertiveness and self-esteem. Many students come to a community college after they have worked in other occupations. They may already be self aware and assertive. They may challenge us by disagreeing with a point we have made. It is always very tempting to dismiss these counterpoints as uninformed or argumentative behavior on the student's part. Our reluctance to have these discussions with students may even stem from some insecurity on our part. It is true that some students use this behavior as adolescents do, as a smoke screen to hide lack of preparation or commitment to the task at hand. However, we should listen and ask the student for a rationale so that we can evaluate their side of the argument. Who ever said that teachers always have to be right? Posing questions to the student should elicit their problem-solving and critical thinking abilities, which can then be redirected. However, *we* may just learn a different view of an area that we thought we had thoroughly explored. The discussion should at least help students to feel respected and empowered.

Many of our students, however, do not ask questions and do not challenge the teacher, but sit passively taking notes and trying to learn the mass of material in a nursing curriculum. We must awaken their ability and willingness to "step up to the plate," to speak out about their thoughts and ideas. If they cannot speak up for themselves, they will never have the courage to be a client advocate. Even the youngest of our students did not drop out of nowhere and into our program. Students come to us with a history, a culture, beliefs, and values. We must help them to use this rich background to believe in themselves. Even if their attitudes and values are contrary to the practices of professional nursing, their views must be acknowledged before they can be changed or used in acceptable ways. I am reminded of a member of the Jehovah's Witnesses who began the nursing course I was teaching with a very confrontational manner and ended it with concrete ways of working within the profession, while staying true to her religious beliefs. We were all enriched by her explanation of these beliefs. It was a given that she could not work in an area that had anything to do with giving blood or blood products but the necessity for her to observe in the operating room as a student was accomplished to the satisfaction of the student and the faculty by using a virtual experience. The student understood the prohibition of proselytizing when the client is in a vulnerable and dependent situation; she could see that this was a form of client abuse and unprofessional behavior, unlike going door to door to preach as a layperson. There are many other examples of students' cultural and religious differences that should be explored privately or in a group so that these beliefs and values can be properly channeled. What remains unsaid cannot be adequately understood and accommodated. We must be willing to be student advocates before we can hope that students will become client advocates.

Once we encourage student assertiveness, we begin the process of interactive learning. We can ask for feedback about difficult concepts after they have been presented. We can ask about students' thoughts and their difficulties with certain topics at the beginning of class. If a particular discussion is getting out of hand or a certain student is monopolizing class time, we can ask that this (these) student(s) see us at the break or after class, or we can challenge her/him to do more research and put it in writing. These strategies usually separate those who just want to challenge the teacher from those with valid points or concerns. Most students in community colleges have little patience for others who waste their class time and appreciate educators who limit discussion to pertinent matters.

Discussions can occur both in class as an interactive approach to learning and/or during clinical conferences. When something occurs clinically that students are concerned about, a clinical conference about all sides of the issue is appropriate at that time. The guidelines for conference topics should be flexible enough to deal with the here and now. After exploring the issues presented, students should be asked to clarify their thoughts about what they would do if they were this client's nurse and what the ramifications or consequences of this action might be for the client, the family, the nurse, and the institution where in took place. Be open to the fact that there may be more than one appropriate solution or no really good, acceptable solution except supporting the client and his family. Faculty should refrain from stepping in to solve the problem, but give information and guidance to help the students think through the issues presented. This approach encourages client advocacy. It also prepares the students for future clinical courses where they will discuss how to help clients and their families explore issues and clarify their values as they struggle with health and/or medical decisions. This, too, is client advocacy.

COLLABORATION AND COLLABORATIVE LEARNING

The above topics all lend themselves to discussion as indicated. What better topic to teach future members of our profession than the fine art of collaboration? Many nurses today find it easier to collaborate with other professionals when caring for patients than to discuss with other nurses the future of nursing. We have witnessed years of conflict within the profession about the level for "entry into practice." There have been many turf wars and a great deal of one-upmanship. With our current and prolonged nursing shortage, we have at least benefited from a more collegial atmosphere as we attempt to attract more students into all nursing programs.

Articulation agreements have become cordial and productive, and it is becoming the norm to value each program and its graduates. Why not start this sense of camaraderie by assigning one of the above-mentioned professional issues for discussion in faculty-chosen groups of two or three students in each nursing course. In each semester, students could focus on any of the ethical or legal issues that are pertinent to their course. See Table 4.1 for a partial list. Students could learn a lot from each other by sharing a common task. This also teaches team-building and consensus-formation skills that are desperately needed in nursing today. Many other fields of study, such as business, have used these strategies for many years because the marketplace demands that their students graduate with these skills. Doesn't professional nursing? We need to go beyond just our program, however. We need to involve students from a practical nursing program, an associate degree nursing program, and a baccalaureate program to help all students in nursing work together. The workplace, the profession, and the future of patient care demand that we graduate students who can work together for a common purpose. It could easily be an objective for students in each program's last semester. It could also be done as a project within the student nurses' association. The results of collaborative work could be a group report either given orally or written. Leadership within the group should be allowed to evolve. It would not surprise me if the student who has more life experiences becomes the project manager, regardless of which nursing program he or she is a member. It goes without saying that the faculty of each program must also demonstrate collegiality and respect for all programs and their students.

NURSING PROCESS AND CRITICAL THINKING

All students are taught the steps of the nursing process and organize their notes accordingly as they learn about various disease entities

and health problems. They must demonstrate their understanding
of the nursing process on tests and in clinical discussions. In most
schools, they must also write care plans. It is a very useful experience
for students to prepare for clinical by doing the assessment and
planning steps, including writing outcomes and outcome criteria by
which the degree of attainment of outcomes can be evaluated. They
learn appropriate interventions to try with the client and hopefully
some scientific rationale for these interventions. This must be viewed
as just the beginning of the process of delivering nursing care. After
working with the particular client for whom the care plan was developed, students further assess and evaluate the planned interventions
to refine and individualize care. Finalizing the care plan and presenting it verbally or in writing helps the student to develop critical
thinking skills. It also helps faculty to evaluate the students' development and how much future assistance each student needs. The
eventual goal is to graduate students who are at a beginning level
of appropriate clinical decision-making in the delivery of nursing
care to individual clients. This "art of nursing" takes practice and
time to ripen, and almost always matures well after graduation. Expectations of generic students in all basic programs must be realistic.
Objectives written for the last semester should not be expectations
of a second semester student. Objectives must be written in each
course that are appropriately leveled to demonstrate student growth
in understanding and their ability to use critical thinking skills.

Brenner, Tanner, and Chesla in *Expertise in Nursing Practice* point
out that nursing students need multiple examples of individuals and
families experiencing what they have learned in class in order to
apply this knowledge. They also need the guidance of an experienced
clinician to help them see the range of human concerns about illness
and suffering, and to understand particular patients' and families'
issues, concerns, and coping strategies. If we take this expanded
view, we can help students to devise more appropriate nursing interventions that individualize patient care. "With openness and willingness to learn from continued experience, experts practice intuitively
rather than through rational calculation in both their understanding
and management of the patient's situation. Students . . . need experience working side by side with an experienced nurse who can point
out salience, nuances and qualitative distinctions" (Benner, Tanner, & Chesla, 1996, p. 308).

Teaching clinical decision-making must start with a theoretical
framework gleaned from the textbook, lectures, and classroom dis-

cussion. After an initial assessment of a client's medical diagnosis and treatment plan and a review of the client's health history and demographics, a clinical prep sheet can be devised identifying relevant data to be used for the clinical experience. Next, the student should be helped to use analytical skills and critical thinking to gather any pertinent missing data and generate possible rationale for this data. Data should not remain just in the physiologic realm, but increasingly should include information gained from interviewing the client and/or family about their fears and concerns, the extent of the knowledge of their condition and what needs they would like the nurse to meet. Clinical faculty and staff need to help the student differentiate between relevant and irrelevant data and begin to formulate a plan of care for a particular client (Su, Masoodi, & Kopp, October–December, 2000). For example, a client on her first postoperative day after a cesarean delivery should be assessed for hemorrhage, fluid and electrolyte imbalances, and pain. The fact that she is not interested in learning about how to care for her new baby at this time is not relevant to her care. If this disinterest persists, then it becomes relevant. Obviously, the more opportunities a student has to care for clients with similar problems, the greater the student's ability to compare and contrast individual needs and the more developed this analytical thinking will become. Students should be provided with a "safe environment in which they can reveal to themselves and the teacher where their knowledge may be limited or lacking and where the clarity of their thinking breaks down" (Benner, Tanner, & Chesia, 1996, p. 323). Without this freedom to ask questions and try out critical thinking skills, clinical judgment will not evolve. I am not saying that we cannot be concerned about some of our students' inability to process information. Of course, if we do not see progress in their critical thinking, we should talk with a student and point out these difficulties. However, if the student fears ridicule and/or an unsatisfactory evaluation from the start, he/she will not be open to these discussions and will constantly try to analyze "what the teacher wants" rather than focusing on learning and developing maximally. We often learn best from our mistakes, but we must be free to make them first within the context of clinical supervision and patient safety. "The impact nursing education has on professional socialization will depend on the students' past experiences, the reflective nature of the process and the beliefs and values promoted in the course" (Howkins & Ewens, 1999).

REFERENCES

Benner, P., Tanner, C. A., & Chesla, C. A. (1996). *Expertise in Nursing Practice.* New York: Springer Publishing Company.

Howkins, E. J., & Ewens, A. (1999, February). How Students Experience Professional Socialization. *International Journal of Nursing Studies, 36.* pp 41–49.

Martin, F., Dall'alba, G., & Beaty, E. (1993). Conceptions of Learning. *International Journal of Educational Research, 19.* pp. 277–330.

Riley, J., & Fry, S. (2000, second quarter). Nurses Report Widespread Ethical Conflicts. *Reflections on Nursing Leadership.* pp. 35–36.

Stabinski, J. (2000, May 22). Ethical Dilemmas: A Systematic Approach. *Advance for Nurses.* p. 7.

Su, W. M., Masoodi, J., & Kopp, M. (2000, October–December). Teaching Critical Thinking in the Clinical Laboratory. *Nursing Forum.* pp. 30–35.

5

How to Motivate Students to Want to Learn

Every teacher must be, in the truest sense of the word, a scholar and an artist. By this I mean one who loves and studies a subject and continually seeks to improve in it. The proper method of teaching a given art is available only to those who, by personally engaging in that art, have become conversant with its inner necessities . . . True teachers not only impart knowledge and method, but awaken the love of learning by virtue of their own reflected love (Grudin, 1990, p. 147).

APPLYING THEORY OF MOTIVATION

In Abraham Maslow's theory of motivation, he describes self-actualization as "the desire for self-fulfillment [and] to become everything that one is capable of becoming" (Maslow, 1987, p. 22). The need for self-actualization only emerges as we each experience some degree of satisfaction of the lower physiologic, safety, love, and belonging and esteem needs (Maslow, 1987). This is true for teacher and student alike.

In order for us, as educators, to be motivated to become "scholars and artists" and to inspire students to love learning, we must feel that our basic needs are met to a great degree and that we are safe at work and in our personal environments. In fact, my first lecture as a full-time faculty member at a community college was on Maslow's Hierarchy of Needs. I had done my research and started to prepare an outline when a particularly violent hurricane threatened the east coast of Virginia. My husband had gone to help his mother secure her coastal property and planned to stay with her during the storm. I was very concerned for their safety and could not seem to progress any further on my preparation for my class. When they arrived at my front door several hours later, I was relieved, and prepared a place for my mother-in-law to sleep. I started writing again. Soon after, my husband's brother and his family, who also lived along the coast, called to ask if they could come. I woke my children and moved them into the same bed so there would be a place for everyone to sleep. Next I was concerned that I would not be able to feed everyone in the morning. At this point, I could not finish preparing my lecture but decided to use this example to explain Maslow's Needs the next day. This may have been the best object lesson I could have used to help students understand the dynamic and fluid nature of this hierarchy. My lecture on this subject was definitely different than any that had ever been presented before.

To a progressively lesser degree, we must experience a connection with those around us. We need to experience self-respect and the respect of colleagues, students, and administrators. If we must constantly justify our job or live in fear that bad evaluations from students will have dire effects on our employment and/or salary, we will not be motivated to question the status quo, dare to try something new, or challenge students to work harder at learning and growing as professionals. This, perhaps, is where faculty with experience can impact positively the careers of newer faculty by supporting their efforts to grow, both individually and publicly. Giving new faculty encouragement and praise for their accomplishments, especially in the presence of administrators and in faculty meetings, would help them feel more comfortable in their new role.

As we attempt to teach this love of learning, we must also remember that not all students come to us ready or willing to self-actualize. Some may fear for their safety or have unmet physiologic needs that mitigate any scholastic effort. This is more fully covered in chapter 6. Some of the qualities of self-actualization that we must teach students, mostly by example, are acceptance of self and others, spontaneity in behavior, compliance with a code of ethics, autonomy rather than conventional thinking, and problem-centered rather than ego-centered behavior (Maslow, 1987). In today's terminology, we must help students to "think outside the box" by doing it ourselves.

In order to motivate students, we must be "user-friendly" and involve them in the creative and interactive process of learning. We can set the stage in the first class by introducing ourselves as "facilitators of learning," stating how they may reach us and giving specific, concrete objectives for our performance and theirs. The more they know about how they will be evaluated, the more secure they will feel in the environment and the better they will understand how they should proceed. If class discussion is expected, then students need to plan and come prepared. A discussion of students' own goals for the course is also important. They may have never before been asked to state their own goals for a course and may need help and some examples to get started. *Their* objectives should also be specific, concrete, and measurable. As important as their goals are, their rationale for these goals are equally worth exploring. This should help the instructor to individualize his/her teaching to the needs and experiences of this particular class. If the class is too large to accommodate most student responses, then we can ask for a show of hands after the more assertive students give their contributions in order to give others a chance to express shared concerns.

A discussion of the knowledge and experiences *they* bring to this course is a good next step to giving the students a sense of progression from one semester to the next, from personal experiences to professional growth. Some students may have the idea that they are starting from scratch with each course, each textbook, each chapter and it is worth the time and effort to remind them that they are not. The task at hand then becomes more doable and students should feel more secure and energized to learn.

How do the students plan to achieve their goals? What is their plan of action? What are they willing to do to achieve their educational objectives? It is probably important at this point to suggest time management strategies that other successful students have used and discuss ways to plan for tests in this course. Some students may need to rethink their strategies and, for example, decide how they are to study at home before their children go back to school in the fall semester. Students with proactive plans should be encouraged to share these with their peers. It might also help to schedule a time for last semester's students to interact with current students.

An additional strategy is to ask students how they will evaluate the achievement of their goals and how often. The students who only use test results may become very discouraged at their "lack of progress," while others who use grades, comfort in the clinical environment, and clinical performance evaluations will balance out their sense of self-growth. Placing the responsibility for learning on the student usually motivates them to move at their own pace and not look for external cues regarding their achievements. Follow-up questions as to how often they plan to take stock of their progress and what they anticipate could interfere with this progress should be asked. If problems can be anticipated then possible solutions can be devised. Suggest to the student that self-evaluation should be done on a weekly basis so that new strategies can be instituted if needed, before it is too late. What if their strategies do not achieve learning objectives? What is their "plan B?" Plan B is an acceptable alternative to a student when plan A is not achievable. Having a plan B tends to decrease anxiety and the "all or nothing" mentality. What can faculty do to help? Sometimes an easing of a deadline, some one-on-one instruction, or even a course incomplete, is warranted, depending on the circumstances. Letting the student know that they are not alone in this learning endeavor very early in the course can make or break his/her success. Obviously students need to be weaned toward self-reliance as the semester and the program of study progresses. Box 5.1 outlines the important issues I have just discussed, to set the stage on the first day of class.

Being an approachable instructor who cares and uses individualized teaching methods does not, however, mean that we should lower standards or change course or program objectives. It simply means that we, as nursing faculty, have to stop expecting RN-level performance until the end of the last clinical course and we must take the time, especially with our nontraditional students, to understand the many stressors in his or her lives and offer compassionate suggestions and advice. To dismiss a potential nurse or future nursing leader as "unworthy" simply because she/he chooses to put his or her young child on the school bus instead of being on time for our 8:00 AM class is nonsense. Helping a student to deal with overbearing and negative parents or in-laws may save a future nursing career. Helping students to build an effective support system will not only pay dividends for the student, but will generate good will and a positive reputation for the nursing program. I have recently read and now recommend to students the book *How to Survive and Maybe Even Love Nursing School! A Guide for Students by Students* written by Kelli S. Dunham (Dunham, 2001). The author is an older student who graduated from an associate degree nursing program and went on to receive her BSN. She is now in graduate school and serves as a shining example of what community college students can accomplish. Her advice will serve students well and provide faculty with

BOX 5.1 **Setting the Stage: First Day of Class**

1. Introductions

   - Shake each student's hand as they enter class
   - Learn students' names and what they wish to be called ASAP
   - Tell students how you wish to be addressed
   - Introduce yourself as a facilitator of their learning.

2. Course Objectives

   - Interactive classes based on discussion
   - Expectation that students will have read material for class
   - Explanation of how this will benefit them

     - More interesting class
     - Increase learning and retention
     - Clarification of information

   - How students will be graded/evaluated.

3. Students' expectations of this course

   - What they would like to learn
   - Personal goals/objectives

     - How will they measure achievement?
     - How often will they take stock?

   - Expectations of faculty

4. What might interfere with their learning?

   - Academically
   - Personally/family/work
   - Time management

5. What if personal goals are not being met at level desired?

     - What is student's "Plan B"?
     - How can faculty help?

insights into the reasons students are having difficulty. It also provides useful advice to share with students. The ability to facilitate student learning is enhanced by a positive classroom environment. Increasing the time given to the course introduction will pay dividends for the rest of the semester and perhaps beyond.

CREATING EXCITEMENT IN THE CLASSROOM

Attitude is everything and a positive attitude is infectious. Expect students to come prepared and conduct class in a manner that rewards those who do. This makes obvious the need to publish specific class topics and not just "module 2" or worse "module 2 continued." Even wording such as "Electrolyte balance made simple" or "What you always wanted to know about diabetes but were afraid to ask" would pique students' interest and make them want to come to class or maybe even read the chapter. Start the class with clear student-centered objectives and explain your plan for helping students meet them. Ask about students' experiences with or concerns about the planned topic. This should encourage even those not prepared to contribute. Take what is offered and use it in some way to give information and explain pictures, diagrams, charts, or other information in the text. Then ask more questions. My philosophy of teaching is that the educator's job is to make the students' reading assignments come alive in the classroom. We need to make dry and complex content memorable.

To aid discussions of pathophysiology, you can use overheads showing pictures, diagrams, and algorithms or you can draw arrows to indicate movement or progression. A video clip showing animation is also a good way to show students how something happens. It might also induce students to view the whole recommended video or CD.

If you are concerned that students are not taking notes, give them a copy of yours or have them download your outline or PowerPoint slides from blackboard or other web-based media. Use your notes to ask students questions, such as "Which assessment data or intervention is most important and why?" Word your questions as the test questions will be worded and tell students that that is what you are doing. They are sure to pay attention. Play "what if" games to take standard answers to a new critical thinking level. And be sure to ask many times, "Why is it important for the nurse to know this?" In more advanced courses, students could be asked to give an example of how they would use the information presented in class in a clinical situation.

Some classes could be constructed ahead of time, so that students plan to teach a specific aspect of nursing care to a classmate, using strategies that would help him or her to retain this information. Pairings could be randomly chosen on the day of class or assigned ahead of time. Mixing the pairs would help to insure fairness and maximize learning. Prior to attempting this strategy, however, it is important to give students many examples of teaching strategies so they have a wealth of options to choose from. Many educators have pointed out that lecture is the least productive method in terms of retention of material. The other, mostly passive learning strategies on which teachers often rely include reading and the use of audiovisual material and demonstration. Much more useful strategies that Sousa describes in *How the Brain Learns* include, in order of increasing importance, discussion, demonstration-redemonstration and teaching others or additional means of immediate use of material. The 24-hour retention rates of such teaching methods are 50, 75, and 90% respectively. Box 5.2 contains a list of instructional methods used, with the average retention rate after 24 hours. The list " . . . devised in the 1960s by the National Training Laboratories of Bethel, Maine (now the NTL Institute of Alexandria, Virginia), comes from studies on retention of learning after students were exposed to different teaching methods" (Sousa, 2001, p. 95). The more active students get into the learning process on their own and in class, the more self-confidence they will have about their knowledge base and the better they should do on tests.

BOX 5.2   Average Retention Rate After 24 Hours

1.	Teach others or immediate use of learning	90%
2.	Practice by doing	75%
3.	Discussion groups	50%
4.	Demonstration	30%
5.	Audiovisual	20%
6.	Reading	10%
7.	Lecture	5%

AROUSING CURIOSITY AND
THE THIRST FOR LIFE-LONG LEARNING

Instructors' energy and enthusiasm about nursing in general and their particular courses, both clinically and in the classroom, go a long way towards motivating students to want to learn. Teaching is often like acting. It is a performance. You must be focused, positive, well prepared, and ready to engage students. Give students your notes, then only use some of them and let students know where you are in your outline. Then ask a lot of "whys" and "what ifs" and "what's the most important information to know about this?" Use PowerPoint slides, if you must, but put the ones that you *really* want to use on overheads, use a CD that allows you to skip around to certain slides or just put certain slides and/or pictures in your slideshow. Slide presentations are very boring if you just read them to the students. And they will never raise their hands if they are busy copying what is on your slides. If you handed out your slides as slides or as an outline ahead of time, then why are you reading them to these students? Haven't you told them that part of preparation is reading your notes and the text? Why should they, if all you do is repeat what they have already done? It will only take one or two classes for students to decide not to come prepared or not to come to class.

So get excited, make eye contact with as many students as possible, move around the room, give humorous examples. A change in facial expression, body language, and voice quality will make an impression and help students to pay attention and remember content. When describing problems with a body part, point to it, diagram it on your body, demonstrate movement. When I teach mechanisms of labor in the maternity course, my shoulders, head, and neck move as the fetus does and my hands form the introitus. When students get to that question on the test, most of them do the same thing. When I teach muscle strength testing in a health assessment course, I demonstrate on my own body or use a student volunteer. Then I ask why this testing is important and when a nurse might need to do this with a client. Don't be afraid to look silly if your goal is to help students remember the monumental amount of information and concepts you are trying to teach.

As an educator, you need to decide whether you are going to teach to the unit test, to the NCLEX blueprint, and/or teach what students need to know to function clinically now and in the future. I personally feel that I need to prepare students for the future by at least introducing new possibilities, therapies, and alternative treatments that clients may ask about or already be using. Students need to be aware of what is "out there" and new ways of thinking about client needs. Just as students must get more involved in their learning process, so also must clients become more involved in understanding their body, nutrition, lifestyle changes, and as much of the ins and outs of their physical and psychological state as possible. In this age of technology and the consumer health movement, clients may have more information than the student. It behooves the student to listen and evaluate the correctness of this information and to help the client apply this knowledge appropriately. Students need to be prepared to ask clients good, appropriate questions and then teach them what they need to know as they give nursing care. We all know that doing discharge teaching on the day of discharge is ludicrous. So why not teach students how to talk to clients and their families about why they are doing what they are doing from their first client interaction? The students and staff will find it easier and more productive to teach the client and/or family how to continue this care at home. When we ask students "why" or "what if" questions, we help them to see the value of thinking more critically. We need to encourage them to use these strategies to teach clients how to stay healthy after discharge.

CHUNKING, REHEARSAL, AND OTHER RETENTION STRATEGIES

The goal of teaching is to help the learner move material into long-term memory. This is critical in nursing, since our graduates must pass a licensing exam and use what they have learned in nursing school to give safe and competent care to future clients. Registered nurses are legally, ethically, and morally accountable for their actions. Their clinical performance and judgment must flow from knowledge and understanding of the science of nursing, as well as from the critical thinking skills that were fostered in nursing school.

Sousa, in his book *How the Brain Learns,* defines retention as " . . . the process whereby long-term memory preserves a learning in such a way that it can locate, identify, and retrieve it accurately in the future" (Sousa, 2001, p. 85). Rehearsal is an important strategy used to retain information in long-term memory. Sousa makes the distinction between rote rehearsal, the storing of information exactly as it entered into memory, and elaborate rehearsal, the processing of new information via previous learning. The latter allows the student to explore similarities and differences, assign value and relevance, and elaborate on the details of the new information (Sousa, 2001). This type of rehearsal is a learned skill and most students need guidance in its development and use. It is the basis for critical thinking and depends on students having read the material to be discussed before class. Strategies for teaching this skill include demonstrating how to elaborate on taught material and then asking students to paraphrase a concept discussed or give an example not mentioned in the book or notes.

Paraphrasing can be done in the margin of the textbook or class notes but it basically should include the statement "In other words, this is saying that . . . " or "what this means is that. . . . " Putting content into their own words helps students to see its relevance and will make it more accessible to them now and in the future. Students should be taught and reminded to ask these questions as they read test questions as well. Ask students to develop higher-level test questions based on the material covered. This not only helps them to prepare for a test, but also encourages deeper thinking by leading them to clarify concepts, make valid associations with prior learning, and apply content to nursing care. Of course, faculty must provide examples of how to write higher level questions at the beginning of the course before students can be expected to continue the process.

Chunking is another means of increasing retention. "Chunking occurs when working memory perceives a set of data as a single item. . . . Chucking allows us to deal with a few large blocks of information rather than small fragments" (Souse, 2001, p. 109). It is analogous to putting many items stored in a computer's hard drive into appropriately labeled files. The information is more logically organized, and it is easier to find and retrieve a certain piece of data if we only have to sort through a few file names, as opposed to large numbers of saved documents. A learner can deal with a great deal more information if taught how to link new items to chunks already in working and long-term memory. Teachers can help students to activate prior knowledge with questions that recall what they already know about the topic of discussion. Prior knowledge can come from personal experiences, general knowledge, or from prior nursing and non-nursing courses. Once an area of interest has been established, discussion about similarities and differences, structure and function, and advantages and disadvantages can make links and expand files already in long-term memory

The degree of retention of new material also depends on timing. Circadian rhythm regulates many body functions, including our ability to focus on incoming information. Studies have shown that for most preadolescents and adults, peak learning occurs between 7:00 AM and 12:00 PM, drops off considerably for the next 20–60 minutes, increases to a lesser peak between 2:00 and 3:00 PM, and is sustained with slight decline as the day and evening progress. Adolescents have their peak, decline, and second peak about an hour or so later in the day (Sousa, 2001). Implications for teaching include the following:

1. Testing during siesta time is probably a bad idea and breaking for lunch is a good one.
2. Afternoon classes should start at 2:00 PM rather than 1:00 PM, the lowest point for cognitive development.
3. Learning attempted during the mid-day trough will require more effort from both the teacher and the student.

Another equally important fact is that we are most attentive and focused on new learning at the beginning third to half of the class period and during the last third, given a 50- to 80-minute learning episode. Studies have demonstrated that the longer the class, the greater percentage of class time is downtime (Sousa, 2001). Implications for teaching include the following:

1. Avoid discussion or questions about content during the first half of the class, when students are primed to remember what is said. Students will remember any incorrect information presented during this time even if the teacher refutes it.
2. Save discussion, questions, practice, or other activities for the middle of the class. This will allow the learner time to organize, process, and use the new material, without adding more new material at a time when retention is most difficult.
3. The last third of the class time is the second most powerful learning time and should be used to help students solidify information given earlier by using chunking techniques of

analysis, synthesis, and evaluation. Ask students to compare and contrast, find similarities and differences, or discuss pros and cons or implications for nursing care.

4. Save announcements for downtime or at the last few minutes of class. Do not waste prime-time educational minutes with details that have little to do with the lesson. Send announcements by email, write them on the board during downtime, or put them on your last slide or overhead if you think you will forget.

5. If the class is longer than an hour, give breaks every 80 minutes or less in order to minimize the percentage of time lost to downtime. Covering more content without frequent breaks is counter-productive.

Chunking and rehearsal techniques take time, energy, and creativity to utilize in class and clinical settings. The rewards, however, include a more energized and thoughtful group of students who are usually better prepared for tests and for nursing practice. Critical thinking is not possible without a sufficient knowledge base stored in the long-term memory and the ability to apply that knowledge to new and different situations. We can tell our students that they should not cram for tests, but unless we teach them alternative ways of attempting to master a large volume of material, they may know no other strategies. This is especially true if cramming has produced good grades for them in the past. Using timing to increase focused learning is worth considering as we organize our class content.

INVOLVING STUDENTS IN SELF-EVALUATION

A colleague of mine successfully achieved funding to provide camcorders for students to videotape themselves doing several procedures in her fundamentals course. After students view their tape, they critique their own performance using a procedural "check-off" form. They have the option to redo the videotaped procedure and critique, or to submit the first video with critique in-lieu of a typical instructor-monitored check-off. The instructor reviews the tape with the student and discusses the student's self-evaluation with concrete suggestions for improvement. Instructors who have participated in this project are amazed at how much insight students gained from evaluating their videotaped performance. Most students are eager to participate in a more-or-less high-tech strategy and seem more relaxed doing the procedure since they can do it over again outside the presence of the instructor. Faculty have found that doing check-offs in this manner takes less instructor-time with almost no need to have the student repeat the check-off. It has increased students' self-confidence and appears to be a win-win proposition.

Another colleague has her psychiatric/mental health nursing students videotape a therapeutic communication project as their first interpersonal process recording (IPR). Each student writes a scenario concerning a depressed client and then role-plays that client. Another student reads the scenario and then interviews the "client" on the videotape. The second student then views the tape and analyzes his/her own therapeutic verbal and non-verbal communication skills. This instructor does not view the tape but looks for student growth and insight from their analyses. If the critique is inadequate, the student does a second tape. The project is done at the beginning of the course and is followed later by a written IPR, done with a client in either an inpatient or outpatient facility. My colleague has found that students are less nervous and more genuine and spontaneous if they know the tape is for their viewing only. They are more able to see non-verbals that are non-therapeutic. This exercise helps students to evaluate how they present themselves to clients, as well as identify areas that need improvement and methods to assess their progress throughout the course and, presumably, their career.

Of course, there are other ways of involving students in self-evaluation. Traditionally, they complete clinical evaluations with comments or examples of how they have or have not met written objectives. In addition, they should summarize their strengths and weaknesses at midterm and at the end of the course. Students could also be asked to generate an action plan to improve areas of weakness. All of this should be done prior to comments written by clinical instructors. Most students will need instructors to give examples and/or guide them on how to proceed, especially in the first two clinical courses. Self-evaluation is part of becoming a professional and maintaining accountability. Introspection also inspires more growth than any external source of evaluation. Students need to be taught to focus as much attention on their strengths as their weaknesses, so they have the self-confidence to change. We, as their teachers, must remember to do the same.

TESTING AND TEST REVIEWS

We must use objective measurement in order to assign a grade. Tests in nursing use higher-level questions than most students have ever experienced before. So we need to help them make the transition, not only with practice test questions but also in how they study and prepare for class. Using "how," "why," and "what if" questions will help them to go beyond the surface. It should also train them to ask themselves these questions as they read textbook information and the teacher's notes. But I think we must do more than this. We must, early on in the curriculum, expose students to Bloom's taxonomy (Sousa, 2001) and indicate how test questions use these higher thinking levels. We must then give examples of the kind of questions we might ask about the information presented. Box 5.3 lists the levels according to the taxonomy with examples of questions written for each level. We can use a handout with questions on it or put questions on a transparency for in-class discussion. A rationale for the right answer must be given. In fact, all of the content could be covered in this manner, by simply discussing the ins and outs of a series of high-level questions. It is absolutely essential that we train our students to take nursing tests if we want them to succeed. They come to us having done well with knowledge level questions in non-nursing courses. They have been "taught" that this is all they need to prepared for their first nursing test. Letting any student flunk their first test as a "reality check" is not part of compassionate teaching. This only enhances resentment, negative thinking, and a sense of powerlessness. If a nursing program, or course faculty within it, feels that only the strong and wise should survive, then they will have a negative impact on the nursing shortage and damage the school's reputation in the community. I have taught a test-taking and learning strategies course for many years and included a brief outline of this course in Box 5.4. The key components of this course include the following:

1.   Use of empowerment and assertiveness strategies
2.   Developing an appropriate support system
3.   Time management techniques
4.   Stress management techniques
5.   Review of reading strategies and study skills
6.   Understanding higher level test questions

BOX 5.3 Examples of Questions Using Bloom's Taxonomy

KNOWLEDGE: Recalling information, repeating information with no changes.

Which of the following ranges represents a normal fasting blood sugar?

a. 60–100 mg/dl
b. 70–110 mg/dl
c. 90–126 mg/dl
d. 110–140 mg/dl

COMPREHENSION: Understanding ideas, using rules, following directions, selection of facts.

You are assessing a client who is taking digoxin. Which statement by the client would indicate that the client may be experiencing toxicity?

a. "Things look yellow and blurry to me."
b. "I have not had a BM in three days."
c. "I hear a ringing in my ears."
d. "I am only urinating a few drops at a time."

APPLICATION: Apply knowledge to a new situation, explaining significance, giving rationale.

You are caring for a client with type 1 diabetes. In mid/afternoon, the client becomes pale and complains of a headache. You should first:

a. take the client's vital signs.
b. administer prescribed insulin.
c. check capillary blood sugar.
d. call the client's physician.

ANALYSIS: Seeing relationships, breaking information into parts, compare and contrast.

You are assigned to a group of clients. Which of the following clients should you assess first?

a. A 19-year-old with septicemia whose first dose of IV antibiotics is infusing and who is complaining of throat tightness.
b. A 25-year-old who had a rhinoplasty 2 hours ago and is complaining of postop pain.
c. A 38-year-old with anemia who has a unit of packed red cells infusing and who is complaining of fatigue.
d. A 69-year-old with emphysema who has a pulse oximeter reading of 92% and is afraid of getting short of breath again.

BOX 5.3 *(continued)*

SYNTHESIS: Putting ideas, information together in a unique way, predict, infer, solve problem.

A client with type 1 diabetes is in her third trimester of pregnancy with her first child. For which of the following bleeding complications would she be most at risk?

a.   Ectopic pregnancy
b.   Placenta previa
c.   Abruptio placentae
d.   Septic abortion

EVALUATION: Making judgments, assessing the value or worth of information.

You have completed teaching for a client with type 1 diabetes. Which statement, if made by this client, would indicate the need for further teaching?

a.   "I can give my shot in the leg and go for a walk."
b.   "I should give my insulin right before I eat."
c.   "I should check my feet for soars at bedtime."
d.   "50% of my calories should come from carbohydrates."

This course is about much more than how to pick the correct answer. Several of these topics are discussed in chapter 6; reading strategies and study skills are covered in chapter 3. Students cannot enroll in the course prior to their first semester in nursing because I have found that they get more out of the classes after they have been exposed to the rigors of a nursing course. It is usually offered a month or so after the first semester begins, or during the summer term. This course is intense and compact, given over a short period of time to quickly maximize its benefits and give students strategies to use right away. Students begin to understand how their own sense of self-worth, use of a support system, sophistication with time and stress management, and reading and studying strategies impact their performance. At the beginning of each class we discuss the strategies each student has started to implement and what benefits they are achieving as a result. Once students realize that they are studying for knowledge-based test questions and nursing questions are at the comprehension level or higher, they understand why these questions are so difficult and in depth. We practice writing higher level questions, using a chapter in their fundamentals text or their health

---

BOX 5.4   **Elements of a Test-Taking Course**

---

1. Discuss of students' analysis of their difficulties with test taking.
2. Use empowerment and assertiveness strategies.

   - Use of body language
   - Use of affirmations
   - Ask for praise from loved ones
   - Do something everyday just for yourself

3. Develop support system.

   - Positive, caring people
   - Avoid negative people

4. Work on time management techniques.

   - What is really important and why
   - What can be delegated
   - What can wait until school breaks or graduation
   - How can you use available time more productively

5. Practice stress management techniques.

   - Levels of anxiety
   - Unique, student specific signs and symptoms of anxiety
   - Simple stress management techniques

     - Deep breathing
     - Progressive relaxation
     - Imagery
     - Music
     - Putting things in perspective
     - Humor
     - Dress rehearsal for test

   - Practice several techniques

6. Review reading strategies.

   - Pre-reading strategies

     - Activate prior knowledge
     - Preview chapter
     - Ask yourself questions about material

   - Strategies during reading

     - Annotate main idea
     - Define new words in margin
     - Restate in own words out loud
     - Visualize what you are reading

BOX 5.4   (continued)

- Post reading strategies

    - Restate main ideas in writing
    - Reduce amount of information
    - Organize information in new way
    - Use information in some way
    - Moves information to long term memory

7. Rethink use of study skills.

    - Come prepared to class
    - Take notes with a purpose
    - Ask yourself questions while actively listening
    - Star areas indicated as important by teacher
    - Review notes as soon as possible after class and correlate with text
    - Have a plan on studying for tests
    - Don't cram
    - Understand information; don't memorize
    - Ask questions about material at comprehension and higher levels
    - Relate new material to prior knowledge
    - Compare and contrast
    - Participate in small study groups

8. Understand test questions.

    - Differentiate case scenario from stem
    - Understand level of question (Bloom's Taxonomy)
    - Identify key words in stem
    - Identify client and issue of stem
    - Decide if stem calls for global or specific answer
    - Read all options
    - Classify options as to true or false statements
    - Eliminate incorrect option or distracters based on above understanding of stem
    - Reread stem to be sure option chosen really answers question in stem
    - Move to next question and don't come back
    - Use educated guesses now not after you have completed the test
    - Do not change answers unless you are absolutely sure.

assessment text. I often use a difficult chapter that most students have not read yet, such as the chapter on fluid and electrolyte balance or assessment of the nervous system. I want them to have a positive commitment to working with the strategies taught, so as to increase their success rate on a future test. The goals have to be tangible to the student. However, not all students can afford the time and expense of an extra course. Therefore, giving examples of test questions in most classes in *every* course remains essential. Our philosophy as educators must lead us to empower students and encourage them to be the best that they can be. Failing even one test does a lot of psychological damage. Prevention is the name of the game, here as well as in health care.

What about test reviews? You know, that masochistic exercise most instructors dread. Well, it doesn't have to be that way. A test review should include the giving and receiving of specific feedback concerning test questions. It is an opportunity to reinforce learning and correct misinformation. It also gives the instructor feedback that will help him or her improve future tests. Was there confusion about test directions or the way a question was worded? The review can also help students evaluate their learning progress, and test taking and study strategies, as well as get help when different strategies are needed. If a test review becomes a battleground between the faculty and the students, then the true purposes are negated and everyone loses. Test reviews conducted in such a manner increase student distrust of faculty and escalate the importance of students fighting for every point. From the educator's perspective, the battle becomes a threat to his/her control over the class. Reviews should be done only after conducting a test and item analysis in an unrushed manner. Students may be given the answers earlier, in a brief and business-like manner at the end of class, but a true test review should be conducted later. If tests are taken on the computer in class or at a testing center, or on-line at home, rationale for the correct answers should be provided. Students can then get instant feedback before possibly reviewing test items in more depth with the instructor at a later date. This is good use of the instructor's time, and still offers students the feedback they want on their performance.

PAPERS AND CARE PLANS

Assessment papers, care plans, research papers, and journal writing should be designed to help the student grow and learn. Another valid use of paperwork is to assist in evaluating students' ability to apply course content, to demonstrate understanding of the nursing process, and to use critical thinking skills. In other words, paperwork can be a very good evaluation tool. However, the rationale for assigning anything that will take a student's time and energy away from studying must be clearly explained. It is best put in writing, along with specific directions and criteria for grading, even if grading is satisfactory or unsatisfactory. Students need to understand if a written clinical project will impact their clinical evaluation. If you want students' best work, sell them on what they will gain from this experience. Paperwork can be constructed to help them pull many areas of the course together or gain depth of understanding by applying course content to a particular client's nursing care. They can learn to evaluate that care and, if stated client outcomes were not achieved, to revise the plan of care. In the case of journal writing, students can reflect on the progress they have made, pose questions, and think "out loud." Journals, however, should be read by the instructor and responded to in a timely manner, and should not be used against a student. If the student is to be honest in this journal, the student must trust the teacher and the teacher must win that trust. There are many uses for paperwork in nursing courses, not the least of which is to give an example of writing across the curriculum. Paperwork is also a way for some students to demonstrate their competence and knowledge base when their test grades may not. The more students derive personally from following explicit directions and understanding the purposes of the paperwork, the harder they will work and the more they will be motivated to learn.

WHY TEACHERS FAIL TO MOTIVATE STUDENTS

There will be some students in any program who are self-starters. They will learn what they perceive as important, no matter how uninspiring the teacher might be. Others, for a variety of reasons covered in chapter 6, will not be successful, no matter what we do as educators. But for the majority of students in any given class, the teacher can make or break their learning experience. These are the students who will be energized and taught to love learning by the variety of methods described in this chapter. Teachers fail to motivate students when they are perceived as unapproachable, don't get to know their students, and don't vary their approach to teaching based on the needs of each particular group they teach.

Don't set your expectations too low. Individualize your approach to students. If they meet course objectives quickly, then motivate them to exceed these with positive feedback and constructive criticism. I have been amazed at how many rise to the occasion. These students are often pleasantly surprised at their own progress and appreciate the vote of confidence that an educator gives when he/ she explains that the student is capable of more. However, with very busy community college students, the option of just meeting expected outcomes must remain. It should be the student's choice whether or not to excel.

There should be multiple options to achieve success in nursing. Objective testing is only one method of evaluating a student's learning. Thought should be given to the use of quizzes that do *not* use a multiple-choice format and the grading of clinical papers with more than a satisfactory or unsatisfactory. Even with clear guidelines, the problem of subjectivity comes into play when there are multiple clinical faculty. If clinical papers are to be given a grade, the following suggestions may be useful. Make papers short enough so that one person can grade them all. This person will also be in a better position to evaluate the clarity of the guidelines, make useful changes, and pick up on duplication of content from student to student. During the semester, a second care plan, teaching project, pediatric play paper, or interpersonal process recording can demonstrate progress and the ability to use feedback. The first attempt should accompany the second if revision of the first is the purpose of this last project. If a grade is assigned, the second paper should count more or be the only one graded in order to encourage students to try harder and follow written feedback. Too many students start from scratch with each project and need to be reminded to build from previous work, even if it is in another semester.

An educator who is truly a facilitator of student learning is user-friendly. Students need to be encouraged to contact the teacher for help with the learning process. If a student has a question about how to proceed and a simple explanation can send him or her in the right direction, why not give it? Learning is not intuitive and the clearest of instruction might become confusing for some students at this time in their lives, for a number of reasons. An invitation by the instructor to call or e-mail questions will encourage trust and empower students to do their best. It goes without saying that feed-back should also be positive and uplifting. It is a lot easier to revise something if the positive points are highlighted, along with what needs to be corrected. Even a smiley face or some other positive sticker is a good tool to motivate adults to do even better.

Teachers who encourage student contact may also discover obsta-cles to success that can be dealt with in a timely manner, prior to a student failing a test or handing in incomplete or unsatisfactory work. Some students simply cannot study for a test and produce good written work in the same week, or when their children are on spring break. Giving the entire class more time to complete the work in such instances should produce better test grades *and* better papers. If a student is taking several other non-nursing courses, listen to their concerns, evaluate the merits of their requests, and act accordingly. Producing competent practitioners, and not setting up roadblocks to success, should be the objective. I have known many students who have done very well in the end, but needed just a little understanding at the beginning or in times of personal and/or family crises.

TEACHABLE MOMENTS

A teachable moment is when someone is ready to listen, change, and grow. We see this with patients who are finally ready to admit that their lifestyle really does have to change after a major illness or exacerbation of their disease process. Students may have teachable moments after they recover from a bad grade or realize the value of maximized learning when they or a loved one needs information that they should have, but do not. A learning principle states that adults learn best if they can see how the information benefits them directly. We need to make these connections for students before they experience a crisis, if possible, by asking pertinent questions. We could ask how they would explain the rationale for diet and exercise to a family member with type 2 diabetes, or what they would think if they were a patient of the nurse who returns from a break smelling of cigarettes. We often use and teach our students to use the learning principles in Box 5.5 when teaching adult clients. Why not use these same principles when teaching our adult students? However, if it takes a "whack on the side of the head" (von Oech, 1998) or a "kick in the pants" (von Oech, 2000) to get a student's

---

BOX 5.5 Learning Principles for the Adult Learner

---

1. Learning occurs only when a person is ready to learn.
2. Learning occurs most quickly if a person can see how new information will benefit him.
3. Adults learn best when new information builds upon preexisting knowledge.
4. Adults learn best when rationales are explained at their cognitive level.
5. People learn best those things that hold particular interest for them.
6. People learn best by active participation.
7. Learning is more likely to take place in a non-stressful and accepting environment.
8. Learning occurs best if rewards not penalties are offered.
9. Learning ability plateaus and time is needed to process information already learned before there is interest and motivation to learn more.

---

attention, seize the motivating moment in a positive and caring manner.

REFERENCES

Dunham, K. S. (2001). *How to Survive and Maybe Even Love Nursing School!—A Guide for Students by Students.* Philadelphia: F. A. Davis Company.

Grudin, R. (1990). *The Grace of Great Things: Creativity and Innovation.* Boston: Houghton Mifflin Company.

Maslow, A. H. (1987). *Motivation and Personality* (3rd ed.). New York: Harper and Row Publishing, Inc.

Sousa, D. A. (2001). *How the Brain Learns, A Classroom Teacher's Guide* (2nd ed.). Thousand Oaks, CA: Corwin Press, Inc.

von Oech, R. (2000). *A Kick in the Pants.* New York: Warner Books.

von Oech, R. (1998). *A Whack on the side of the Head: How You Can Be More Creative* (3rd ed.). New York: Warner Books.

6

Why Students Fail and What to Do About It

> *Higher needs require better outside conditions to make them possible. Better environmental conditions (familial, economic, political, educational, etc.) are all more necessary. . . . Very good conditions are needed to make self-actualizing possible* (Maslow, 1987, p. 58).

Despite our best efforts to help students, some will not pass our courses for a variety of reasons. The second part of the survey which was mentioned in chapter 3, dealt with professors' assessments of factors which contribute to poor performance of students in the first and second years of the nursing program (Box 6.1). My purpose here was to see which areas persisted in the last two semesters and to compare the data from this survey with a similar one (Box 6.2) done with students who were taking a test-taking course. Students in this test-taking course are usually self-referred or referred by faculty for help in improving grades. I have not included any data from the students' survey since the number of students was too small to be significant. I plan to add to this data survey results from students in future classes as well as ask all students to take this survey.

As in the faculty survey of teaching strategies, I received some additional contributing factors that faculty members thought should be included. I have included the expanded list in Box 6.1 and suggest that faculty members use it to evaluate admission requirements and plan remediation strategies. This should increase the number of students admitted that are ultimately successful in completing the nursing program in a timely manner, and, more importantly, in passing the RN licensing exam on the first try.

Obviously, most faculty members felt that poor academic, reading, and study skills; working too much; and coming to class unprepared

---

BOX 6.1   Faculty Survey of Causes of Student Difficulties
in Associate Degree Nursing Programs

Please rate according to the following scale and differentiate between 1st &
2nd year:

1   do not agree   2   agree somewhat   3   agree   4   strongly agree

In my opinion many nursing students have difficulty in the nursing curriculum
because they:

		1st year	2nd year
1.	Have poor academic preparation	____	____
2.	Have poor English skills	____	____
3.	Have poor math skills	____	____
4.	Work too many hours	____	____
5.	Do not spend enough time studying	____	____
6.	Consistently come to class unprepared	____	____
7.	Have no experience in nursing	____	____
8.	Lack sufficient educational equipment at home (books, computer, nursing journals, etc.)	____	____
9.	Lack financial resources to acquire what they need	____	____
10.	Lack a significant support system	____	____
11.	Have family that active provide blocks to success	____	____
12.	Lack self-esteem	____	____
13.	Lack reading and study skills	____	____
14.	Lack test-taking skills	____	____
15.	Lack critical thinking skills	____	____
16.	Have personal or family health issues	____	____
17.	Choose nursing for the wrong reasons	____	____
18.	Are not committed to being the best that they can be	____	____
19.	Need college facilities to be available when they are able to use them (weekend, evenings, etc.)	____	____

Please add any other assessed characteristics of students that, in your opinion, impair learning and success in nursing.

---

were deterrents to success in the nursing curriculum. Programs can
counter some of these factors by identifying students with academic
weaknesses using college placement tests and NLN pre-admission
test scores and providing appropriate remediation and re-testing.
Many community colleges offer a basic study skills and orientation
to college course. This course should be mandatory for all students

BOX 6.2   Student Survey of Learning Difficulties in Associate Degree Nursing Programs

Please rate according to the following scale:

1 do not agree   2 agree somewhat   3 agree   4 strongly agree

I am having difficulty in the nursing curriculum because I:

1. Have poor academic preparation   _____
2. Have difficulty with English   _____
3. Have difficulty with math   _____
4. Work too many hours   _____
5. Do not spend enough time studying   _____
6. Consistently come to class unprepared   _____
7. Have no experience in nursing   _____
8. Lack sufficient educational equipment at home (books,   _____
    computer, nursing journals, etc.)
9. Lack financial resources to acquire educational material   _____
10. Lack a significant support system   _____
11. Have family that actively provide blocks to success   _____
12. Lack self-confidence   _____
13. Lack reading skills   _____
14. Lack study skills   _____
15. Lack test-taking skills   _____
16. Lack critical thinking skills   _____
17. Have personal or family health issues   _____
18. Have difficulty understanding English vocabulary   _____
19. Have difficulty understanding medical terminology   _____
20. Have difficulty understanding most instructors   _____
21. Do not keep up with reading assignments   _____
22. Do not use practice test questions to prepare for tests   _____
23. Have uncontrolled anxiety during the test   _____
24. Do not understand my learning style   _____
25. Need college facilities to be available weekends, evenings   _____

Please circle whichever applies: I am having difficulty in classroom, clinical/LAL, or both.

Please add any other difficulties that have made learning and success in nursing more difficult for you.

Please indicate in which semester you are currently enrolled. _____

beginning their college experience. It should also be a prerequisite to applying to any curricular program. Those planning to request admission into the nursing curriculum should be offered additional guidance as to the importance of non-nursing courses, such as anatomy and physiology and English composition, to the success of their nursing studies.

Not all students who wish to participate at the college level have the necessary ability to master the rigors of the nursing program. Providing information sessions each semester to prospective students, outlining the expectations of the nursing curriculum, the time commitment, and the sacrifices that this might entail would help students to be more realistic. Having current students give examples of how they have had to organize their lives might give credence to the advice. Showing a factual video of a day in the life of a nurse might deter those who are looking at a nursing career as just a job. Increasing the number of scholarships and financial aid packages for qualified students might ease the need for some students to work full time, as would providing health insurance policies at group rates.

What surprised me most in the survey was how often faculty teaching second year students rated the above issues, as well as poor test taking and critical thinking skills, at a 4 for their students who were not doing well. How have students with these deficits and problems moved to this level without correcting them? How will they complete the program of study and pass the licensing exam? What are we as educators doing to help students overcome these deficiencies? These are questions that deserve our attention. I have included a discussion of many of these areas in this chapter. Basically, a caring teacher needs to make time to discuss with each student who is having difficulty, the following areas of possible concern: any current life crises, how they feel about themselves, evaluation of their support system, allocation of their time, evaluation of study and test taking skills, and any conflicts between teacher and student expectations.

STUDENTS EXPERIENCING CRISES

A person's trust and capacity for growth can be limited by unmet fundamental physiologic and psychosocial needs. In the process of self-actualizing, reality has a way of derailing the most motivated individuals. Although crises can happen to anyone, community college students may be more vulnerable and often have less financial and personal reserves to help overcome life-changing events.

When a person's ability to provide food and shelter for self and family is threatened, he/she may have to drop out of school to work full time. The injury or death of a parent, wife, or husband who provides financial support, or a perceived or real threat to personal and/or family safety can dramatically shift a student's ability to focus on academic pursuits. These issues are not easily overcome in the short term. Faculty can offer support by listening, asking open-ended questions, perhaps assisting the student in formulating a plan of action. We can refer them to particular school counselors with expertise in grief support or abuse counseling. In addition, we can inform students of procedures for withdrawing from classes without academic penalty. We can also submit a "withdrawal for mitigating circumstances" if the drop date has passed. When warranted, an incomplete grade can be given if a student will be able to complete a project or a final exam in the not-too-distant future. We should give the student information about the process for reapplying to the nursing program when his or her life is more stable. Most of all, we should listen and praise them for taking stock of their situations and attempting to take control. Some students may need our "permission" to withdraw and use their energies to solve the more basic problem of surviving the crisis at hand. They may feel like they have failed to live up to their potential or to our expectations. I have often reminded them of Maslow's hierarchy of needs, and how motivation to self-actualize is not possible when their more basic needs are threatened.

Some students facing the above circumstances may continue in our classes, with no possibility of success. They continue to dig their academic holes deeper and deeper, because they are not aware of their options. They may not trust faculty to help or understand, perhaps because of negative experiences with past teachers. A good teacher can spot a student in turmoil and must make every effort to reach out to that student. Do not wait for the student to approach you. Teachers must often take the first step and then help these students to use more effective critical thinking and assertiveness skills. Allowing a student to self-destruct without trying to intervene is not the action of an effective educator. A student may or may not take the advice given, but a caring professional has to try.

FEAR OF FAILURE

Success may be over-rated and may induce complacency. However, an occasional failure can be a wake up call, a humbling experience, and can lead to a "teachable moment." Failure tends to put things in perspective, allowing us to rethink our priorities, our definition of success, and our strategies for the future, that is unless our "successes" are few and our "failures" are many. So it is important that we ask those students who are not doing well in our program to define both success and failure and to describe their strengths to us verbally and then in writing. I am always amazed by how difficult this seems to be for struggling students. I try to get them to describe themselves by asking questions. I ask, "What is it about yourself that makes you most proud?" Most talk about their children or their family, but not their contributions that have enhanced others' success or their own successes. I ask, "What skills and talents do you bring to nursing?" Many will list caring, hard work, and desire to help others, but not their interpersonal skills. I ask, "What academic successes have you experienced in the past?" Even though all students must have achieved at least a C or better in nonnursing courses to be accepted into the nursing curriculum, students who are not doing well in nursing tend not to remember these successes, nor to use them as encouragement.

When students define themselves as failures, it will become a self-fulfilling prophecy. Many come from families that have helped them to feel negatively about their ability to succeed. Some suffer from an all-or-nothing, perfectionistic view of life. If the grade is not an A, then it is a "failure" in their eyes, and sometimes in the eyes of those who constitute their support group. Negative reinforcement from self and others can tear away at even the most optimistic and self-confident student. Students who are struggling tend to have lower self-esteem and engage in negative and demeaning self-talk. We also cannot forget the secondary gains of such behavior. Students who "know" they are going to fail a test and then do so usually get a lot of support from peers and often from instructors. We are, after all, caring people. Do those who do well get this same support? What effect does the expectation that a student, who usually does well, will get an A on each test have on that student? What a lot of pressure! In the eyes of some students, playing "poor me" is a choice they make, even if it is subconscious. Their avoidance of the expectation of success may be as strong as their fear of failure. Some students may need counseling to deal with these underlying issues.

We can point our students who simply suffer from test anxiety in a different direction. Early on in the program, most students learn about the physiology of the fight-or-flight mechanism. We can help them to remember the physiologic manifestations of anxiety and identify those signs and symptoms that they experience *first*. We can simulate a test-taking situation and have them list their symptoms. They can then practice slowing their respiration and pulse rate with deep breathing exercises. Progressive relaxation can lower blood pressure and induce a feeling of calm and control. Learning such techniques and using them at the first sign of anxiety can empower students to take control of their situation. They must also start to use self-affirmation and learn to verbally and physically pat themselves on the back and accept praise from others. Then they can be encouraged to ask members of their support system to say or do certain things that will help them think more positively about themselves. Teaching children to "give Mom a hug" because she needs a lift will not only be therapeutic for the student, but also will teach the child interconnectivity and increase the child's self esteem. Once a student can see how asking for help from family and friends also benefits those asked, they are more willing to do it. Books like *Taking the Anxiety Out of Taking Tests: A Step by Step Guide* by Susan Johnson (Johnson, 1997) are inexpensive and easy to read and follow. Campus bookstores should stock them.

LACK OF OR NEGATIVE SUPPORT SYSTEMS

You can choose your friends, but not your relatives. However, you can choose how often and when you interact with them. Appropriate support systems are very important to all of us, but they are crucial in times of stress. As faculty, we need to ask about students' support systems. A student having difficulty may or may not realize that relatives and friends may be sabotaging their efforts at being success-ful. Students often relate that their significant others refuse to help around the house or with the care of children. Worse yet, they may cause the student to feel guilty for not being able to do what he/she did prior to nursing school. They often make plans without consulting the student about the timing of tests and papers. If a student is not doing well, family members may make them feel stupid or incompetent, which only increases the student's sense of failure and hopelessness. Some of these students even choose friends who are sarcastic and demeaning, as if that is all they deserve. Teachers can be instrumental in helping students to understand the detrimental nature of these encounters with the very people they should be able to count on for support. Some students already realize this, but need help in formulating an action plan to counteract the unwanted input from negative people in their environment. Permission to tell in-laws not to visit until the semester ends may be just the empowering strategy a student needs to turn his or her grades around. Helping a student to word a plea for help and respect from a significant other or a parent may also be all that is needed. All too often, however, the problems are significantly more involved, and students need to be referred to a school counselor who deals with such issues. A list of agencies that deal with physical or psychological abuse should be in every faculty member's drawer. The percentage of abused women in any college, but particularly in community colleges, would surprise many. As these women try to better themselves and improve their economic situation, their significant others, who usually do not have a college education, may feel threatened. His subtle and not so subtle sabotage of her study time may take the form of constant interruptions and requests for her time, or refusal to help with childcare and household chores. Criticism of her efforts in school and outside of school is often a spouse's ploy to discourage a student, even when she is doing well. Derailing her efforts by compromising their financial situation by taking out a new car loan or a new mortgage, or financing the purchase of furniture or a dream vacation may prevent her from cutting back on her work hours. She may find herself being talked into an ill-timed pregnancy that further complicates her struggle to be successful.

WOMEN'S ISSUES

In addition to the above-mentioned abuse and negative support issues, women in general seem to have needs that must be overcome in order for them to be successful in their studies. This is especially true of nontraditional older students, who have families and a job and are active members of their communities. They have difficulty saying "no" to requests from family members, their bosses, co-workers, their church, and others. The very traits that potentially make them good nurses, such as caring dispositions, strong work ethics, and good assessment and planning skills, threaten to derail their success in school because everyone counts on them for help. These students find it easier to put their own needs last. Students often need help in viewing their situation realistically. They may need encouragement to find ways to redirect those who ask for their help. We can also empower them to ask for and accept help from others. As students progress through the nursing specialties, it is easier to use object lessons about co-dependency and enabling behavior to show them that they might help others more by *not* taking care of things. Convincing a student to hold their children accountable for behavior in and out of the home, and to expect them to do age appropriate chores gets easier as the student matriculates through pediatric nursing.

Some women may also feel helpless, as if they have no realistic options, if they continue to fail test after test. At least we can help them to decide to withdraw from the course before it affects their GPA such that they are unable to return to the program. They may need time to grow and learn from the experience of poor scholastic performance. We can help them to explore alternatives to the RN program, which may be more doable in their present circumstances. I have had the privilege of teaching students who returned to the associate degree program after achieving success in an LPN program. Their current skills, understanding of nursing, and self-esteem were remarkably improved, which made their success in the nursing program *this time* much more likely.

MEN'S ISSUES

Women are not the only students with issues and with families that may sabotage their efforts to get an education. Men may feel the need to remain the primary financial provider, even when this results in lack of study time and failing grades. This can be compounded by their significant others, who may convince them that they need a bigger house, a better automobile, or that the timing is right to have a child. He may be made to feel guilty because he is not as responsible in the partnership as he was, because he is not as much fun as he used to be, or because he is neglecting her and/or their children. In too many instances, male students have dropped out of nursing and higher education without seeking help or explaining their circumstances with a teacher. I now make it a habit to talk with students who do not do well on the first test. I do not wait for them to make an appointment with me, since I know that some never will. Early discussion of potential problems with male students who have failed the first test may help them to generate solutions that would not be as useful later in the semester. In addition, men in nursing must often justify their choice of profession to family and friends. Nursing is still seen as woman's work and is less valued than medical school. Men who choose nursing school need to be encouraged to seek out other male nurses for support and encouragement (MED-ZILLA.com, June 6, 2002). Their unique perspective on issues that may only confront men in the field cannot be provided by female nurses and faculty. I frequently refer male students to the American Assembly for Men in Nursing through their e-mail address at *aamn@aamn.org* and to *www.MinorityNurse.com*. However, times are changing. I rarely have patients refuse the care of a male nursing student, even in labor and delivery, but that was not always the case. Also, staff nurses now judge male students more by their character and work ethic than by their gender.

POOR READING, STUDY, AND ACADEMIC SKILLS

With pre-entrance testing and appropriate remediation, this is less of a problem than it once was. However, with nontraditional students, nothing can be assumed. Depending on the degree of difficulty the student is having, a teacher may be able to help by offering a few study tips, referring a student to an academic support center, buddying the student with a willing classmate or someone from a prior class, or referring the student to a Math or English teacher who is willing to help. Academic support centers are essential in community colleges, since the student population comes from such diverse backgrounds. There are federal and sometimes state grants available to finance such centers and to pay recommended student tutors. This support center should be able to advise students with diagnosed learning disabilities in a variety of learning strategies that make sense.

  If academic difficulties are appropriately dealt with in the first semester, they should not persist in future courses. If students are not able to read at the 10th grade level or do basic math, then how can they pass the fundamentals of nursing course? We cannot, especially in this time of cut-backs in higher education, expect a fundamentals instructor to counsel all beginning students by herself. Beginning students need the most experienced faculty and the smallest faculty-to-student ratio. Adjunct faculty cannot fill this gap. It would be helpful if faculty who usually teach upper level courses teach at least one module in the nursing fundamentals course. This can help faculty members learn to simplify the content, as they teach beginners. It will also show them how far students have come when they arrive in their upper level courses. Furthermore, it familiarizes the students with faculty they will meet in the future, begins the faculty-student relationship, and makes it more likely that students will feel comfortable approaching all faculty with questions and concerns. Since I have been teaching some content to first semester students, students view me as user-friendly and approachable. I can also remind them of what they have learned in the past and help them to apply those concepts to new material. Faculty can teach other concepts such as time-management, study skills, and test-taking strategies discussed in Chapters 3 and 5. If we provide appropriately for the basic nursing education and advising of beginning students, we will improve retention rates and provide the guidance that students need to remain successful throughout the program and as professional nurses. Our students may well be our best recruitment strategy for nursing in general, and for our program in particular, if we respect them and help them in their studies, regardless of whether or not they are successful. They can also do great harm to the recruitment efforts if we treat them badly. This thought should give us all something to consider.

PROCRASTINATION AND TIME MANAGEMENT

Waiting until the last minute to do something difficult is part of human nature. Most of us learn the hard way that this is not a good strategy for success. Some of us persist in using it, nonetheless. I have always started my test-taking course by passing out a weekly schedule for students to fill out, starting with those items they have no control over, such as work, class, and clinical times, commuting times, eating and sleeping times, and any other fixed scheduling items. Then I ask them to fit in class/clinical preparation and study times. I suggest a ratio of two to four hours per hour of class and two to four hours pre-clinical preparation time. When some students do this, they find that there are not enough hours in the week to handle all they have taken on, and that fact is driven home without a word from me. Cutting back on work or getting someone else to do children's car pools, grocery shopping, meal preparation, etc., becomes an obvious necessity. I ask them to finalize their schedule once they discuss it with family members and return it the next class day. This is a homework assignment for which they receive points. I then suggest that they post the completed schedule for all to see, and train family members to refer to it by pointing to it whenever anyone asks them to do something extra. Students consistently tell me that this it is one of the most useful strategies they learned in the course. When they follow their schedule, they come prepared to class and allow sufficient time to look up medications, treatments, and medical diagnoses prior to clinical. They tend to be more comfortable in class and clinical, and do not need to cram for exams. This strategy works much better than a lecture on time management. My second strategy in teaching time management is to suggest that they always have a Plan B. And when they are using Plan B, a Plan C needs to be developed. This is also a very effective stress management tool, and students usually find it very useful. I use both strategies when counseling individual students, as well; however, they miss the class discussion with input from others. There are, of course, some students who are unable or unwilling to put these strategies into practice. Some students are so over-committed that they cannot possibly be successful at something as time-consuming as nursing without a major overhaul of their lifestyle and priorities. For them, I suggest that it may not be the best time to attend nursing school.

RIGHT BRAIN THINKERS IN A LEFT BRAIN WORLD

The left and right hemispheres of the human brain are distinctly specialized and process information differently. Dr. Roger Sperry of the California Institute of Technology won the 1981 Nobel Prize for medicine in part for his work in charting the characteristics of each hemisphere and identifying the purpose of the corpus callosum, the thick cable of nerve fibers that connects the two hemispheres and allows for the sharing of memory and information between the two (Sousa, 2001). Information about the right and left hemispheres and its uses for teaching and learning are, therefore, relatively new. When we think of those who mostly use their left brain, we consider them to be more logical thinkers. They are analytical and organize factual data in a rational manner. They are time and sequence sensitive. The speech center is in the left hemisphere and it recognizes words, letters, and numbers as words. The right brain, on the other hand, is the intuitive hemisphere. It interprets language through tone of voice, emotional content, and body language, as opposed to literal meaning. Right brain thinkers are spatially sensitive and focus on faces, objects, places, and music. They process information more holistically and abstractly than left-brain thinkers (Sousa, 2001). Hemispheric preferences contribute to learning style.

Most people are left brain thinkers. Most nurses, faculty, and nursing students are left brain thinkers. But the right brain visionaries we have the privilege to meet, enrich our lives and our practice. Nonetheless, a right brain student in nursing school sticks out like a sore thumb, as does a right brain teacher. Getting them together is very helpful to both. The rest of us are left to teach a creative, spatially and intuitively oriented student how to "critically" think in an orderly, linear, step-by-step manner. Why? Encourage students to come up with creative ways of remembering concepts and prioritizing interventions, and then ask them to share these with the class. Use pictures and illustrations from the textbook to make a point and help both right- and left-brain students remember. Move around the room and use sweeping gestures to illustrate behavior or nursing activity. Most of us are visual learners, no matter which side of our brain is most active.

Mind mapping is a particularly useful learning strategy for right brain students and helps them to remember relationships and sequences of activities. It also moves a right-brain student from the general idea to specific pieces, from the big picture to subordinate ideas using key words (Ellis, 2000). It is much better for these students than taking notes. Taking the time to show a student how to do this, or referring the student to a study skills text may turn his difficulties into successes. Helping a student to understand that we may think in different ways, but that neither way is better is also important. Helping left-brain students to understand a right-brain teacher may be more difficult. Giving these students a detailed set of notes and then providing a dramatization of the content is a very useful strategy for such teachers. Left-brain students will be frustrated with such activity, however, without the notes. When students learn to take the best that any teacher has to offer and interpret the material in their own special way, then long-term memory is enhanced and learning has been achieved.

POOR TEST TAKING SKILLS

Teaching students the levels of Bloom's Taxonomy and giving examples of test questions that use these levels is one of the best ways to help a beginning student understand why nursing tests are so difficult. Refer to Box 5.3 for specific examples. As I have said before, this should be done in the first semester and perhaps repeated at the beginning of the second semester. In my test taking class, students can see the difference between various questions and begin to focus more on exactly what the stem of the question is asking. They learn to recognize a comprehension question and can distinguish between a question that requires analysis and one that requires synthesis of information. They can even write their own test questions at the various levels, with a little help. These activities help them learn to read and study differently, so they are better prepared to answer more in-depth questions on tests. Test taking is a skill that can be taught and learned to enhance performance. When students understand that nursing tests are constructed to better prepare them for the NCLEX-RN exam and also to help them function better as a nurse, they begin to accept the need to learn how to work with this format.

Since most students come to us having done fairly well in nonnursing courses, they may resent the fact that they are not achieving the grades to which they have become accustomed. They may state, "I am an 'A' student," so there must be something wrong with the tests that nursing faculty write. The above example of the use of Bloom's Taxonomy (see examples in Box 5.3) usually helps students to change their unrealistic expectations of making A's on all of our tests and helps prepare them to study more effectively.

WHAT TO DO WITH STUDENTS WHO FAIL

Not all students who apply to the nursing program will be successful. We can, as concerned faculty, use the strategies outlined in this and previous chapters to guide students in their quest for success. This may not be enough for some students, however. If we are aware of behavior or incidents in class or clinical that are contributing to a student's lack of success, we can write a contract with the student, listing specific actions the student must take or behaviors that must be avoided in order to pass the class or clinical. I have outlined what should be in such a contract in Box 6.3. Some students may give an unsatisfactory clinical performance that precludes their passing the course, even if their theory grade is high. A contract or some notification of unsatisfactory performance should have been written and signed by the student prior to the end of the term, so that due process is established. I have included a sample student contract in Box 6.4. We must be honest with students in our evaluation of their clinical and classroom performance. Every evaluation should list positive accomplishments, as well as unsatisfactory behaviors. Help students focus on what was well done, as well as on what is preventing them from completing the course. Give them a copy of the evaluation, so they can read it when they are less emotionally involved. Invite them to write a rebuttal of a clinical evaluation if they disagree with it. This rebuttal should be attached to the evaluation. Doing this in the student's presence is very therapeutic and decreases the likelihood of future confrontations. Asking them to complete surveys

---

BOX 6.3   Elements of a Student Contract

1.   Briefly list situations necessitating contract.

   • Behaviors and incidents noted with dates and circumstances surrounding incident.
   • Student's response to discussion about incident.

2.   Specific detailed list of what student must do or avoid doing with due dates, if applicable. (Make each item a reasonable expectation of any student in the class with reasonable due dates—can extend after final exam.)
3.   Consequences of not accomplishing all of items on list.
4.   Signature of faculty with date
     Signature of student with date
5.   Give student a copy and put one in student's school folder. The end result of the contract should be written in the student's folder and clinical evaluation tool, if applicable. If contract has consequences for clinical performance, it should also be attached to the clinical evaluation tool.

BOX 6.4 **Sample Student Contract**

Date _____   Course #_____

This contract with _____(student's name)_____ is being written as a result of
the following behaviors observed during this student's _____(semester in which
behavior occurred)_____ semester in nursing school.

1. _____(student's name)_____ has been late for clinical on
    _____(date)_____ , _____(date)_____ , _____(date)_____ , and late for class on
    several occasions. Behavior has continued despite several one-on-one
    discussions with the student about tardiness.
2. _____(student's name)_____ was unable to discuss several medications
    prior to administering to client on _____(date)_____ demonstrating lack
    of clinical preparation. This behavior was repeated on _____(date)_____
    despite a reprimand after the first incident. The student was dismissed
    from clinical this time.

Contract between _____(student's name)_____ and _____(instructor's
name)_____ .

For the remaining portion of this semester, _____(student's name)_____ will:

1. be on time for all classes.
2. be on time for all clinicals.
3. be appropriately prepared to answer questions about medications to
    be given to client as to dose, route, timing, and purpose of medication
    for this client, common side effects and nursing considerations.
4. be appropriately prepared to administer any treatments ordered for
    clients assigned to him/her as to purpose of treatment and proper
    procedure.
5. participate knowledgeably in clinical conferences and meet all other
    clinical objectives of this course as stated in the syllabus.

If the student cannot meet any and all of the objectives stated above, the
student will receive an unsatisfactory clinical grade and a grade of D (or F)
for the course.

Signatures:

_____(instructor's signature)_____   Date _____

_____(student's signature)_____   Date _____

academic stressors than students in a four-year college. However, based on a current situation at the University of Arizona, the problems and potential solutions that I have covered in this chapter may be more generic to all beginning students than I previously thought. According to an MSNBC News report, a 40-year-old male student who was failing his nursing course entered the room where his midterm exam was being given on October 28th, 2002. He then shot and killed the two nursing faculty members present, as well as a faculty member in another room, before taking his own life. He had previously been tied to a bomb threat against the nursing building (MSNBC, 10/28/2002). These are all extreme and desperate acts of an individual who may have seen no way out of his academic and career difficulties. Are there other potentially volatile situations in the making across our campuses? Who knows? With compassionate concern for them as individuals and not just as failing students, I suspect that we should, *and will*, get better at discerning and working with troubled students, so as to redirect their energies and dispel their sense of isolation and hopelessness. What ever happens after this incident, we as a community of nursing educators have had our own wake-up call. We need to do a better job with students who are having difficulty.

REFERENCES

Ellis, D. (2000). *Becoming A Master Student* (9th ed.). New York: Houghton Mifflin Company.

Johnson, S. (1997). *Taking the Anxiety Out of Taking Tests; A Step-by-Step Guide.* Oakland, CA: New Harbinger Publication, Inc.

Maslow, A. H. (1987). *Motivation and Personality* (3rd ed.). New York: Harper & Row Publishers, Inc.

MEDZILLA.com. (2002, June 6). "Why Are There So Few Male Nurses?" *http://www.medzella.com/press61102.html* 10/4/02.

MSNBC staff and wire reports. (2002, October 28). Four Die in Arizona College Shooting. MSNBC Breaking News. *http://www.msnbc.com/news/827110.asp?cp1=1* 10/28/02.

Sousa, D. A. (2001). *How the Brain Learns, A Classroom Teacher's Guide* (2nd ed.). Thousand Oaks, CA: Corwin Press, Inc.

7

Teachers as Mentors

For these [effective community college] faculty, teaching is more than an occupation; it is a dedication to leave the world a better place; an opportunity to make a difference in another's life; a chance to enhance one's own life through a kind of immortality, that of remembrance (DuBois, 1993, p. 467).

What does it take to be an effective nursing educator in a community college nursing program? Glen DuBois summarizes his research findings in the quote above. He states that the best community college teachers have "a strong command and organization of their subject" and spend a considerable amount of time preparing each class. They present their material with enthusiasm and are "talented in clarifying difficult subject matter." He further states that these effective faculty members are student-focused, approachable, and accessible to their students. They have the desire and ability to motivate their students to work at achieving academic success by frequently evaluating, guiding, and encouraging them. Effective teachers understand that "many community college students come from troubled family experiences and lack academic skills" (DuBois, 1993, p. 463), and never embarrass or berate these students because of their deficits. Effective educators make students like these want to put forth the intense effort needed to overcome their academic and sociocultural adversities, and excel in their chosen field. What a tall order! Those of us who have chosen to teach nursing in a community college setting must, in my view, accept this challenge and work toward becoming the best that we can be. Our students deserve no less.

As faculty members, we can work with peers to make sure that our program remains student-friendly, positive, and accessible, without sacrificing quality and standards. After all, we want all of our graduates to become licensed to practice nursing and to have a rewarding and productive career. If we limit access to our program with pre-admission testing, then we must provide avenues of remediation. Students who have academic deficiencies can learn or relearn math, English, and science skills to improve their performance on these tests. In our classes we must use language and interpretations of content that has meaning to every student. We must be willing to get to know students in order to better advise and nurture them. We must be good role models in our own academic pursuits and share with them our struggles toward excellence. Many of the best teachers have experienced their own academic and personal disappointments and challenges. The more we relate to and with our students, the more they may be encouraged by the fact that we have overcome obstacles, as well.

A PRAGMATIC APPROACH TO MENTORING

Mentoring as defined by Vance and Olsen, "is a developmental, empowering, and nurturing relationship extending over time in which mutual sharing, learning, and growth occur in an atmosphere of respect, collegiality, and affirmation" (Vance & Olsen, 1998, p. 5). Other less formal descriptors of a mentor include role model, counselor, advocate, confidante, advisor, and one who encourages and inspires another (Klein & Dickerson-Hazzard, 2000). I prefer the latter definition, since it opens up more possibilities and does not have to be an exclusive relationship with one person or one that occurs over a long period of time. Many more students and peers can be affected by a caring, affirming professional. I agree with Vance and others who assert that the mentor benefits from the relationship as much as the protégé, experiencing personal and professional satisfaction while observing the growth of another in the nursing profession. Personal and professional development occurs from the intellectual and psychosocial challenges posed by the protégé. Opening oneself to another by mutually sharing stories, insights, and experiences results in learning, growth, and change for the mentor just as much as the person who is mentored. Students often see nursing from a different perspective than nursing faculty, and, when given the opportunity, respect, and encouragement, ask challenging and diverse questions that may stimulate research in

Springer Publishing Company

101 Careers in Nursing

Jeanne M. Novotny, PhD, RN, FAAN,
Doris T. Lippman, EdD, APRN, CS,
Nicole K. Sanders, and
Joyce J. Fitzpatrick, PhD, RN, FAAN

Few careers offer the advantages of nursing: flexibility, room for growth, satisfaction from helping others. And there is a desperate need for nurses; demand will exceed supply for some time to come.

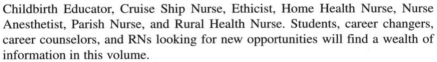

This concise volume provides an overview of what's possible in a nursing career. It profiles 101 different types of nursing careers, including a basic description, education requirements, skills needed, compensation, and related web sites and professional organizations. Personal stories from the practicing nurses highlight the content.

The authors provide information on careers as diverse as Acute Care Nurse Practitioner, Armed Services Nurse, Childbirth Educator, Cruise Ship Nurse, Ethicist, Home Health Nurse, Nurse Anesthetist, Parish Nurse, and Rural Health Nurse. Students, career changers, career counselors, and RNs looking for new opportunities will find a wealth of information in this volume.

Contents:

- Introduction, *J.M. Novotny, J.J. Fitzpatrick, and D.T. Lippman*
- 101 Career Descriptions (including interviews)
- Launching Your Career Search, *T. Robert*
- Notes from My Interview Experiences for a First Nursing Position, *N.K. Sanders*
- Guide to Certification in Nursing
- Glossary of Career Acronyms

2003   240pp   0-8261-2014-8   soft

536 Broadway, New York, NY 10012 • (212) 431-4370 • Fax (212) 941-7842
Order Toll-Free: 877-687-7476 • Order on-line: www.springerpub.com

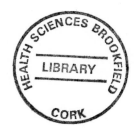
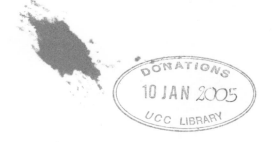